C000179933

Bread Machine Cookbook: 2 Books in 1

Get Fit, Maintain Health, and Save Your Cooking Time with This Amazing Guide About Bread Machine Containing 40+ Nutritious, Mouth-watering and Time-saving Bread Recipes.

© Copyright 2021 - All rights reserved.
The content contained within this book may not be reproduced, duplicated or transmitted without direct written permission from the author or the publisher. Under no circumstances will any blame or legal responsibility be held against the publisher, or author, for any damages, reparation, or monetary loss due to the information contained within this book. Either directly or indirectly.

Legal Notice:
This book is copyright protected. This book is only for personal use. You cannot amend, distribute, sell, use, quote or paraphrase any part, or the content within this book, without the consent of the author or publisher.

Disclaimer Notice:
Please note the information contained within this document is for educational and entertainment purposes only. All effort has been executed to present accurate, up to date, and reliable, complete information. No warranties of any kind are declared or implied. Readers acknowledge that the author is not engaging in the rendering of legal, financial, medical or professional advice. The content within this book has been derived from various sources. Please consult a licensed professional before attempting any techniques outlined in this book. By reading this document, the reader agrees that under no circumstances is the author responsible for any losses, direct or indirect, which are incurred as a result of the use of information contained within this document, including, but not limited to, errors, omissions, or inaccuracies.

BREAD MACHINE RECIPES FOR BEGINNERS

BREAD MACHINE COOKBOOK FOR BEGINNERS

BREAD MACHINE RECIPES FOR BEGINNERS

Table of Contents

INTRODUCTION

Bread Machine Benefits

Tasty custom made bread!

You can make new bread every day. Not any more semi-old store bread that has been sitting in your cooler for quite a long time.

Bread making is simple and straightforward with a bread machine.

No plying... by you. The bread machine accomplishes the difficult work and massages the bread batter for you.

It is a lot speedier than making oven-heated breads. You simply gather the ingredients and add into the bread machine... and sit back until the bread machine is finished. Interestingly, with numerous oven-heated breads, you should invest energy manipulating, trusting that the bread will rise, and plying once more, and so on

No abnormal synthetic or additives. You add the ingredients so you know precisely the thing are going into your family's bread.

You can make custom made breads to coordinate with your family's extraordinary eating routine necessities (for example egg free bread).

Extraordinary for incompetent cooks or cooks with restricted time.

There is no compelling reason to go out looking for sandwich bread during a snowstorm or rainstorm to make the upcoming school snacks. This is an immense advantage in the event that you live in the open country and the closest store is 30+ minutes away.

1. Bread Machine Jalapeno Cornbread (with Cheese)

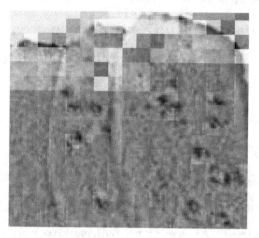

Prep Time: 10 mins| Cook Time: 1 hr. 40 mins | Total Time; 1 hr. 50 mins

Ingredients

- 1 Cup Milk
- 8 Tablespoons Unsalted Butter (mollified)
- 2 Eggs (delicately beaten)
- 1/2 Cups Yellow Cornmeal
- 1 Cup All-Purpose Flour
- 2 Tablespoons White Granulated Sugar
- 3 Teaspoons Baking Powder (aluminum free)
- 1 Teaspoon Salt
- 1/4 Cup Jalapenos (diced into little lumps)

- 1/2 Cups Shredded Cheddar Cheese

Guidelines

1. Unplug the bread machine and eliminate the bread skillet.

2. Dice the jalapenos into little pieces. FYI - You will add the jalapenos after you added the wet ingredients to the bread skillet.

3. Relax the spread in a microwave.

4. Softly beat the eggs.

5. Add milk, margarine, eggs and afterward the remainder of the ingredients into the bread container. Attempt to follow the request for the ingredients recorded above so fluid ingredients are set in the bread container first and the dry ingredients second. FYI - Be mindful that the bread dish ought to be eliminated from the unplugged bread machine before you begin to add any ingredients. This assists with trying not to spill any material inside the bread machine.

6. Spot the bread container back into the unplugged bread machine and afterward plug in the bread machine.

7. Enter the bread machine settings (Quick Bread, Light Color, 2 lb.) and press the beginning catch. FYI – Before making this formula, kindly read the tips area beneath for more data with respect to the "fast bread" setting used to make cornbread. This setting can be confounding on some bread machines... however the tips area beneath will assist you with tracking down the correct setting to use on your machine. You need to enter the right cornbread setting utilized by your SPECIFIC bread machine model or the cornbread could be under or over cooked.

8. At the point when the bread machine has wrapped up heating the cornbread, unplug your bread machine. Eliminate the bread dish and spot the bread skillet on a wooden cutting board. Allow the bread to remain inside the bread search for gold minutes before you eliminate it from the bread dish. Use oven gloves while eliminating the bread container since it will be extremely hot!

9. In the wake of eliminating the cornbread from the bread skillet, place the bread on a cooling rack. Use oven gloves while eliminating the

bread. Allow the cornbread to chill off for 60+ minutes or it will be bound to break/disintegrate when cut into cuts.

10.   Remember to eliminate the blending paddle on the off chance that it is stuck in the bread. Use oven gloves as the blending oar could be hot.

2. Bread Machine - Multigrain Bread Recipe

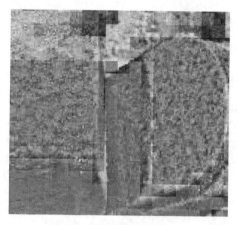

Prep Time: 10 mins | Cook Time: 3 hrs. | Total Time: 3 hrs. 10 mins

Ingredients

- Multigrain Bread - 2 lb. Version
- 1/2 Cup Milk (warm)
- 4 Tablespoons Unsalted Butter (mollified)
- 3 Cups Bread Flour
- 1 Cup Multigrain Cereal
- 1/3 Cup Brown Sugar (stuffed cup)
- 1/2 Teaspoons Salt
- 1/2 Teaspoons Bread Machine Yeast

- Multigrain Bread - 1.5 lb. Version
- 1/8 Cups Milk (warm) - 1/8 cups of milk is identical to 1 cup and 2 tablespoons of milk
- 3 Tablespoons Unsalted Butter (mellowed)
- 2 1/4 Cups Bread Flour
- 3/4 Cup Multigrain Cereal
- 1/4 Cup Brown Sugar (stuffed cup)
- 1 Teaspoon Salt
- 1 Teaspoon Bread Machine Yeast

Directions

1. Bread machine settings – 1.5 or 2 pound portion, light tone and "fundamental" bread setting.
2. Relax the spread in your microwave.
3. Know that the bread skillet ought to be taken out from the bread machine before you begin to add any ingredients. This assists with trying not to spill any material inside the bread machine. The bread machine ought to consistently be unplugged while eliminating the bread container.
4. Empty the milk into the bread container and afterward add different ingredients. Spot the bread machine yeast in last and the yeast

ought not to touch the fluid or salt (until the bread machine is turned on and the ingredients begin to be combined as one).

5. A few groups like to make a little "divot" on top of the flour to hold the yeast in one spot before the machine begins.

6. Put the bread container (with the entirety of the ingredients) back into the bread machine, close the bread machine top and afterward plug in the bread machine.

7. Enter the right settings (for example 1.5 lb. or 2 lb. portion, light tone and essential bread setting) and press the "start" button.

8. At the point when the bread machine has wrapped up preparing the bread, unplug the bread machine. Eliminate the bread from the bread dish and spot the bread on a cooling rack. Use oven gloves while eliminating the bread machine compartment (bread dish) as it will be hot!

9. In the wake of eliminating the bread, remember to eliminate the blending paddle on the off chance that it is stuck in the bread. Use oven gloves as the blending oar will be hot emerging from the bread machine. Or on the

other hand stand by until the bread is totally cooled and afterward eliminate the blending paddle.

10.   In our Sunbeam bread machine, the heating requires around 3 hours for a 2 pound bread portion (and 2:53 hours for a 1.5 lb. bread portion) at the light tone and fundamental bread settings. Nonetheless, a few machines can contrast and you would prefer not to be away from home when the bread machine "completed" caution goes off! Your bread machine should show you the length of the heating time after you have entered the settings into the machine. This will permit you to realize that when will generally be in the kitchen to eliminate the bread.

11.   Prior to utilizing your bread machine, you should peruse the bread machine producer's guidelines to utilize the bread machine successfully and securely

3. Oatmeal Bread Recipe (Instant Yeast)

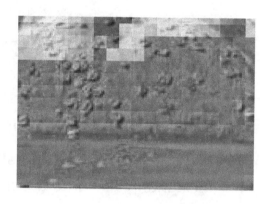

Prep Time: 2 hrs. 45 mins | Cook Time; 40 mins|
Total Time; 3 hrs. 25 mins

Ingredients

- 1/2 Cups Milk (tepid)
- 4 Tablespoons Unsalted Butter (mollified)
- 3 Cups Bread Flour
- 1 Cup Old Fashioned Oatmeal
- 1/3 Cup Light Brown Sugar (stuffed cup) - If you lean toward non-sweet oats breads, you should utilize just 2 tablespoons of earthy colored sugar.

- 1/2 Teaspoons Salt
- 1/2 Teaspoons Instant Yeast

Directions

1. Directions - Creating Dough with a Bread Machine
2. Your bread machine ought to be unplugged.
3. Eliminate the bread dish from the bread machine (so when you add the ingredients, they cannot incidentally spill into the machine).
4. Empty the milk into the bread container and afterward add different ingredients. Spot the moment yeast (bread machine yeast) in last and the yeast ought not to touch the fluid (until the bread machine is turned on and the ingredients begin to be combined as one by the bread machine). A few pastry specialists like to make a little indent on top of the flour to keep the yeast from spilling into the fluids or blending in with the salt before the machine is turned on.
5. Put the bread skillet with ingredients back into unplugged bread machine.

6. Plug in bread machine. Enter the "Mixture" setting on your bread machine and afterward press the "Start" button.

7. At the point when the bread machine has wrapped up making the bread batter, unplug the bread machine.

8. Eliminate the bread skillet from the bread machine.

9. Presently go to the guidance segment beneath on "setting up the batter and heating the bread". FYI - Ignore the guidelines for the electric stand blender beneath on the off chance that you are utilizing a bread machine to make your batter. Skirt down to the getting ready mixture area.

Directions - Creating Dough with an Electric Stand Mixer with Dough Hook

1. Your electric blender ought to be unplugged.

2. Eliminate the blending bowl from the electric blender.

3. Supplement a batter guide into the electric blender.

4. Empty the milk into the blending bowl and afterward add different ingredients. Spot the

moment yeast in last and the yeast ought not to touch the fluid (until the electric blender is turned on and the ingredients begin to be combined as one). A few pastry specialists like to make a little indent on top of the flour to keep the yeast from spilling into the fluids or blending in with the salt before the machine is turned on.

5. Spot the blending bowl once more into the electric stand blender.

6. Plug in the electric blender and utilize a low speed to blend the batter. Blend the batter for 8-10 minutes.

7. Mood killer the electric blender and unplug machine.

8. Eliminate the blending bowl from the electric blender. Empty the batter into a subsequent enormous blending bowl that has been daintily "lubed" with olive oil, liquefied margarine, cooking shower, and so on

9. Freely cover the bowl with saran wrap and let the batter ascend for an hour.

10. After the batter has risen, go to the guidance area beneath on "setting up the mixture and heating the bread".

Directions - Preparing the Dough and Baking the Bread

1. Preheat the oven to 350 F.
2. Sprinkle a tad of flour onto a huge cutting board.
3. Eliminate the batter from the bread container or blending bowl and spot the mixture on the cutting board.
4. Press down on the mixture with your hands and make a "flattish" square shape with the batter. The batter ought to be around 1 inch high.
5. Fold up the batter into a tight "jam roll". FYI - Please see this short instructional video for more data on the best way to shape the batter in the event that you haven't formed bread mixture previously. It is simpler to watch and gain from this short video as opposed to attempting to clarify the moving strategy bit by bit.
6. Optional - If you need to make more "bona fide" cereal bread outside appearance, you can brush a limited quantity of egg white, milk or water on the highest point of the batter with a baked good brush. You will at that point roll

the highest point of the mixture in some oat pieces that you have sprinkled on a cutting board (see picture above) or delicately press some oat chips into the highest point of the batter (which will be tacky because of the egg white/milk/water).

7. Spot the folded up mixture into the bread skillet.

8. Optional - If you didn't fold oat pieces into the highest point of your mixture, you should brush liquefied spread on top of the batter (after you have put it in the bread dish) with a cake brush.

9. Freely cover the highest point of the bread container with cling wrap. Put the shrouded bread dish in a safe spot for an hour for the batter to ascend into a pleasant portion shape. The mixture should rise marginally over the highest point of the bread skillet after this hour long period.

10.   Spot the bread container in the (preheated) oven to heat at 350 F for 37-42 minutes. Wear oven gloves when managing a hot oven. Spot the bread skillet in the oven

11. Turn the bread dish in the oven following 15-20 minutes (to guarantee an in any event, sautéing of the bread). Wear oven gloves.

12. After the 37 brief heating time frames has completed, eliminate the bread dish from the oven. Wear oven gloves.

13. Eliminate the bread from bread skillet and spot the bread on a wire cooling rack. Wear oven gloves.

14. Optional - If you didn't fold oat chips into the highest point of your batter, you can utilize a baked good brush to brush dissolved spread on top of the bread. This ought to be done well after you have eliminated the bread from the bread skillet. This spread "treating" assists with making a more brilliant and delicious hull.

15. Permit the bread to chill off on the wire cooling rack for 1-2 hours prior to cutting the bread.

4. Onion Bread Recipe

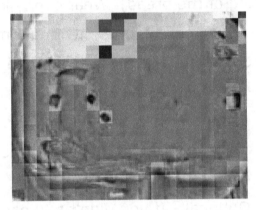

Prep Time: 10 mins | Cook Time; 3 hrs. | Total Time; 3 hrs. 10 mins

Ingredients

- 1 Cup Milk (tepid)
- 4 Tablespoons Unsalted Butter (mellowed)
- 3 Cups Bread Flour (not generally useful flour)
- 1/2 Large Onion (diced and seared)
- 1 Tablespoon White Granulated Sugar
- 1 Tablespoon Onion Powder
- 1/2 Teaspoons Salt
- 1/2 Teaspoons Bread Machine Yeast

Directions

1. Bread Machine Settings - Basic, Light Color and 1.5 lb.

2. Dice the onion half into little lumps. Sauté in a griddle with a modest quantity of spread or vegetable oil until brilliant earthy colored.

3. Mellow the spread in your microwave.

4. Empty the milk into the bread container first and afterward add different ingredients. Spot the bread machine yeast in last and the yeast ought not to touch the fluid, salt or hot sautéed onions (until the bread machine is turned on and the ingredients begin to be combined as one by the bread machine). You can make a little opening or trench in the highest point of the flour and spot the yeast in this opening to keep the yeast separate for the salt, and so forth

5. Plug in the bread machine. Enter the right settings (essential, light tone and 1.5 lb.) and press the "start" button.

6. At the point when the bread machine has wrapped up preparing the bread, you ought to unplug the bread machine. Eliminate the bread and spot it on a cooling rack. Use oven gloves while eliminating the bread machine compartment (bread portion skillet) as it will be exceptionally hot!

7. In the wake of eliminating the bread, remember to eliminate the blending paddle in the event that it is stuck in the bread. Use oven gloves as the blending oar will be hot emerging from the bread machine. Or on the other hand stand by until the bread is totally cooled and afterward eliminate the blending paddle.

8. Prior to utilizing your bread machine, you should peruse the bread machine producer's guidelines to utilize the bread machine viably and securely.

5. Banana Bread Recipe (Classic Version)

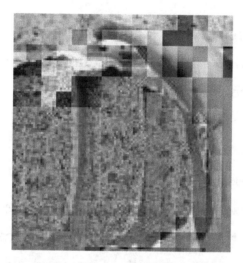

Prep Time: 10 mins | Cook Time: 1 hr. 40 mins | Total Time: 1 hr. 50 mins

Ingredients

- 8 Tablespoons Unsalted Butter (mellowed)
- 2 Eggs (gently beaten)
- 1 Teaspoon Vanilla Extract
- 3 Bananas (ripe and medium-sized bananas)
- 1 Cup Light Brown Sugar (pressed cup)
- 2 Cups Flour (universally handy)
- 1/2 Teaspoon Salt
- 1 Teaspoon Baking Powder (aluminum free)

- 1 Teaspoon Baking Soda
- 3/4 Cup Chopped Walnuts or MINI Chocolate Chips (optional)

Guidelines

1. Planning Time – 10 minutes
2. Heating Time – 1:40 hours
3. Bread Machine Settings – Sweet Quick Bread, Light Color, 2 lb.
4. Beat the eggs.
5. Squash bananas with a fork.
6. Relax the margarine in microwave.
7. Add the eggs, margarine and bananas into the bread dish and afterward add different ingredients. Attempt to follow request of the ingredients recorded above so fluid ingredients are put in the bread skillet first and the dry ingredients second. Know that the bread container ought to be eliminated from the bread machine before you begin to add any ingredients. This assists with trying not to spill any material inside the bread machine. The bread machine ought to consistently be unplugged while eliminating the bread dish.

8. Put the bread dish (with the entirety of the ingredients) back into the bread machine, close the bread machine cover and afterward plug in the bread machine.

9. Enter the bread machine settings (Sweet Quick Bread, Light Color) and press the beginning catch. FYI - Before making this formula, kindly read the tips segment beneath for more data in regards to the sweet speedy bread setting used to make banana breads. This setting can be confounding on some bread machines... however, the tips area beneath will assist you with tracking down the correct setting to use on your machine. You need to enter the right banana bread setting utilized by your SPECIFIC bread machine model or the banana bread could be under or over cooked.

10.   Optional - If you need to add chopped pecans or smaller than expected chocolate chips to upgrade this fundamental banana bread formula, if it's not too much trouble, add them after the principal bread machine blending cycle and before the subsequent blending (last blending).

11.   At the point when the bread machine has wrapped up heating the bread, unplug the bread machine, eliminate the bread container and spot it on a wooden cutting board. Use oven gloves while eliminating the bread container since it will be hot!

12.   Optional - Use a long wooden stick to test if the banana bread is totally cooked. Wear oven gloves as the bread skillet will be hot. See the tips segment for additional subtleties on this exemplary "toothpick" test.

13.   Subsequent to eliminating the bread container from the bread machine, you should allow the banana to bread stay inside the warm bread skillet on a wooden cutting board for 10 minutes (as this completes the heating interaction) before you eliminate the banana bread from the bread dish. Wear oven gloves.

14.   Following 10 the moment "cool down", you should eliminate the banana bread from the bread container and spot the banana bread on a wire cooling rack to complete the process of cooling. Use oven gloves while eliminating the bread.

15.   Remember to eliminate the blending paddle on the off chance that it is stuck in the bread. Use oven gloves as the blending oar could be hot.

16.   You ought to permit the banana bread to totally cool prior to cutting. This can require as long as 2 hours. Something else, the banana bread will break (disintegrate) all the more effectively when cut.

6. Bread Machine Breadsticks (Soft & Chewy)

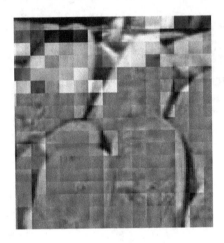

Prep Time: 1 hr. 40 mins | Cook Time: 12 mins | Total Time: 1 hr. 52 mins

Ingredients

- 1/4 Cups Water (tepid)
- 2 Tablespoons Olive Oil
- 3 1/2 Cups Flour (universally handy flour or bread flour)
- 1 Tablespoon White Granulated Sugar

- 1/2 Teaspoons Italian Herb Seasoning (optional)
- 1 Teaspoon Salt
- 2 Teaspoons Bread Machine Yeast
- 1 Teaspoon Large Crystal Salt (to sprinkle on top of the breadsticks prior to heating)

Guidelines

1. Spot the water, olive oil and afterward the remainder of the ingredients into the bread skillet. You can make a little indent on top of the flour to keep away from the yeast falling into the water (until the machine begins). Try not to join the salt with the yeast (as the salt can execute the yeast). Spot the yeast and salt in discrete pieces of the bread skillet.

2. Spot the bread container (with ingredients) into your unplugged bread machine and afterward plug in the machine.

3. Put your machine on the Dough setting and press the beginning catch. In our Sunbeam bread machine, the plying and ascending on the batter setting requires about roughly 1:30 hours.

4. At the point when your bread machine has completed, unplug the machine and pour the mixture onto a cutting board. Wear oven gloves when taking care of the bread skillet as it very well might be hot. In any case, first sprinkle some flour on the cutting board (before you pour the mixture) to help keep the batter from adhering to the cutting board.

5. Preheat oven to 400 degrees F.

6. Shape the breadstick mixture by one or the other cutting into flimsy strips or folding into meager cylinders. See the tips segment underneath for more data on the most proficient method to shape your breadsticks.

7. Spot the mixture breadsticks onto a nonstick heating sheet. Cover them freely with cling wrap, wet meager towel, and so on to keep dust off and to keep the mixture from drying out. Allow the mixture to ascend for 30 minutes on the preparing sheet. The mixture should generally twofold in width during this time.

8. After the mixture has risen and before you put the preparing sheet in the oven, utilize a little cake hedge to cover the highest point of every

batter breadstick with a slim layer of olive oil. At that point sprinkle some huge salt gems (for example ocean salt or coarse genuine salt) on top of every mixture breadstick.

9. Spot the heating sheet in the oven for 12-15 minutes.

10.   Eliminate from the oven when completed and allowed the breadsticks to cool for 1 or 2 minutes on a cooling rack.

11.   For best outcomes, serve and eat while the breadsticks are still somewhat warm.

7. Bread Machine Cranberry Raisin Bread Recipe

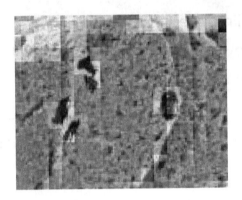

Prep Time: 5 mins | Cook Time: 3 hrs. | Total Time: 3 hrs. 5 mins

Ingredients

- 1/2 Cups Water (warm)
- 4 Tablespoons Unsalted Butter (sliced and mellowed)
- 3 Cups Bread Flour
- 1 Cup Old Fashioned Oatmeal
- 1/3 Cup Light Brown Sugar
- 1/2 Teaspoons Salt
- 1/2 Teaspoons Bread Machine Yeast

- 4 Tablespoons Dried Cranberries
- 4 Tablespoons Golden Raisins

Directions

1. Bread machine settings – 2 pound portion, light tone and "fundamental" bread setting.
2. Unplug the bread machine and eliminate the bread dish from the bread machine. This forestalls any ingredients added to the bread dish from accidently spilling into the bread machine.
3. Beginning with the water, you should add the entirety of the ingredients (aside from the cranberries and brilliant raisins) into the bread machine "pail" (bread container).
4. Spot the bread skillet back into the bread machine and plug in the bread machine.
5. Enter the right settings into the bread machine (for example 2 pound, light tone and essential) and press the beginning catch.
6. After the bread machine has completed its initially massaging cycle (and before the second manipulating cycle), add the cranberries and brilliant raisins.

7. At the point when the bread machine has wrapped up preparing the bread, unplug the bread machine. Eliminate the bread and spot it on a cooling rack. Use oven gloves while eliminating the bread machine compartment (bread portion skillet) as it will be hot!

8. Subsequent to eliminating the bread, remember to eliminate the blending paddle in the event that it is stuck in the bread. Use oven gloves as the blending oar will be exceptionally hot emerging from the bread machine. Or then again stand by until the bread is totally cooled and afterward eliminate the blending paddle.

9. In our Sunbeam bread machine, the heating requires around 3 hours for 2 pound bread at the light tone and essential bread settings. In any case, a few machines can vary and you would prefer not to be away from home when the bread machine "completed" alert goes off! Your bread machine should show you the length of the preparing time after you have entered the settings into the machine. This will permit you to realize that when generally will be in the kitchen to eliminate the bread.

10. Prior to utilizing your bread machine, you should peruse the bread machine producer's directions to utilize the bread machine adequately and securely.

8. Bread Machine French Bread

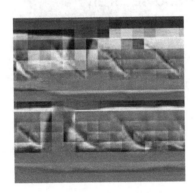

Prep Time: 2 hrs. 40 mins | Cook Time: 20 mins | Total Time: 3 hrs.

Ingredients

- 1/3 Cups Water (tepid)
- 3 1/2 Cups Bread Flour
- 2 Teaspoons Bread Machine Yeast
- 1 Teaspoon Salt
- 2 Tablespoons Olive Oil (to cover batter)

Directions

1. Spot the water and afterward the remainder of the ingredients into the bread dish. You can make a little indent on top of the flour to stay away from the yeast falling into the water (until the machine begins). Try not to

consolidate the salt with the yeast (as the salt can murder the yeast). Spot the yeast and salt in isolated pieces of the bread dish.

2. Put your machine on the "Batter" setting and press the beginning catch. In our bread machine, the working and ascending on the batter setting requires about 1:30 hours.

3. At the point when your bread machine has completed, unplug the machine and pour the batter onto a cutting board. Wear oven gloves (as the bread dish/bread machine might be hot). Sprinkle some flour on the cutting board (before you pour the mixture) to keep away from the batter adhering to the cutting board.

4. Separation the batter into 4 equivalent parts in the event that you need to make 4 thin loaves (about 12 inches in length). Or then again partition the batter into 2 equivalent parts to make 2 thicker French bread "rolls".

5. Roll the partitioned mixture with your hands into your favored shape (for example loaf or thicker bread roll). See our tips underneath on forming the bread mixture (particularly about the making the batter move around 1/2 the

width of your ideal final result... as the mixture extends as the yeast rises).

6. Spot the formed batter onto a nonstick preparing sheet.

7. Coat the mixture with olive oil. Utilize a little cake brush.

8. Cover the batter and heating sheet with a light kitchen material or saran wrap to shield from dust, and so forth

9. Allow the batter to ascend for 60 minutes.

10. During this "rising" time, preheat your oven to 450 degrees F.

11. After the hour, eliminate the covering from the mixture and "score" (cut) the highest point of every batter move with a sharp blade. Make corner to corner cuts around 1/2 inch down and around 3 inches separated. This will help keep the bread from breaking during heating. See the tips underneath about how to score bread.

12. Spot the preparing sheet in the oven. It ought to heat at 450 degrees for 15-20 minutes or until brilliant earthy colored. Wear oven gloves.

13.   At the 8 brief imprint, turn the preparing sheet around to guarantee an in any event, "caramelizing" of the bread. Wear oven gloves.

14.   Eliminate the preparing sheet when done and place the bread on a cooling rack. Wear oven gloves.

9. Bread Machine Italian Bread

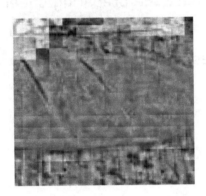

Prep Time: 2 hrs. 45 mins | Cook Time: 20 mins | Total Time: 3 hrs. 5 mins

Ingredients

- 1/4 Cups Milk (tepid)
- 2 Tablespoons Olive Oil
- 3 1/2 Cups Bread Flour
- 1 Teaspoon White Granulated Sugar
- 2 Teaspoons Bread Machine Yeast
- 1 Teaspoon Salt
- 1 Teaspoon Dried Rosemary (Optional - for families who like rosemary-type Italian breads)
- 1/8 Teaspoon Coarse Salt (Optional - sprinkle a touch of salt on top of the batter "portion" not long prior to preparing)

Directions

1. Unplug the bread machine.
2. Eliminate the bread container from the bread machine. Empty the milk into the bread container and afterward add the remainder of the ingredients (with the exception of optional coarse salt). Put the bread dish once again into the unplugged bread machine.
3. Plug in the bread machine. Select the "Batter" setting and press the "Start" button on your bread machine.
4. At the point when your bread machine has completed, unplug the machine and pour the batter onto a cutting board. Wear oven gloves (as the bread container/bread machine might be hot). Sprinkle some flour on the cutting board (before you pour the mixture) to stay away from the batter adhering to the cutting board.
5. Make either 1 huge portion or 2 medium-sized portions (by slicing the mixture down the middle). Shape the batter so it would appear that a semi-restricted (American) football or fat torpedo. See tips segment for seriously forming data. FYI - The mixture roll(s) ought to

be around 1/2 of the width of your ideal completed heated bread width (as the batter will extend prior to being put in the oven).

6. Spot the molded batter onto a nonstick preparing sheet.

7. Coat the batter with olive oil. Utilize a little baked good brush.

8. Cover the mixture and preparing sheet with a light kitchen material or saran wrap to shield from dust, bugs, and so forth

9. Allow the mixture to ascend for 60 minutes.

10. During this "rising" time, preheat your oven to 450 degrees F.

11. After the hour, eliminate the covering from the mixture and "score" (cut) the highest point of every batter move with a sharp blade. Make 3 corner to corner cuts around 1/4 - 1/2 inch down and around 3-4 inches separated. This will help keep the bread from breaking during heating.

12. Optional - Sprinkle a spot of course (salt with huge gems) on the highest point of the oil-shrouded mixture.

13. Spot the preparing sheet in the oven. It ought to prepare at 450 degrees F for 17-20

minutes or until brilliant earthy colored. Wear oven gloves.

14.   At the 8 brief imprint, turn the preparing sheet around to guarantee an in any event, "searing" of the bread. Wear oven gloves.

15.   Eliminate the preparing sheet when done and place the bread to chill off on a cooling rack. Wear oven gloves.

10. Sweet Potato Rolls

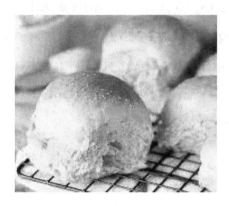

***Prep: 20 mins | Cook: 22 mins | Total: 42 mins
| Servings: 24 servings***

Ingredients

- 2 medium yams (1 cup, crushed)
- 3/4 cup milk
- 3 tablespoons spread (dissolved, in addition to extra to finish rolls out of the oven)
- 1 huge egg (beaten)
- 4 cups generally useful flour (18 ounces)
- 4 tablespoons sugar
- 1 teaspoon salt
- 2 1/4 teaspoons dynamic dry yeast

Steps to Make It

1. Accumulate the ingredients.
2. Strip 2 medium yams and cut them into 3D shapes.
3. Heat a pot of salted water to the point of boiling over high warmth.
4. Add the yam blocks to the bubbling water and diminish the warmth to low. Cover the skillet and cook for around 20 minutes, or until delicate.
5. Channel well and pound.
6. Cool totally and measure 1 cup for the formula.
7. Add all ingredients to the bread machine in the request recommended by the producer.
8. Utilize the essential batter cycle. At the point when the cycle completes, remove pieces from the batter to make balls, and spot in a lubed 9-inch square preparing dish so they're simply contacting yet not very close. (around 1 3/4 ounces each to get around 24 rolls)
9. Cover the rolls with a material and let ascend for around 45 minutes in a warm, without draft place.
10. Preheat oven to 375 F.

11. Heat in the oven for around 20 to 23 minutes, until pleasantly seared.
12. Brush the tops with liquefied or mollified margarine while they're hot.
13. Appreciate!

11. Argentinian Ring Bread

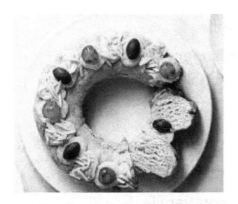

Prep: 4 hrs. | Cook: 45 mins | Total: 4 hrs. 45 mins | Servings: 8 servings

Ingredients

- For the Cake:
- 3/4 cup entire milk
- 2/3 cup sugar, isolated
- 1 tablespoon dynamic dry yeast
- 1 to 2 teaspoons vanilla
- 2 eggs
- 4 cups universally handy flour, isolated
- 1 teaspoon salt
- 1 tablespoon lemon zing (from 1 lemon)
- 8 tablespoons (1 stick) unsalted margarine, cut into pieces

- 1 egg yolk (for egg wash)
- For the Pastry Cream:
- 1 cup milk
- 1 egg
- 1 egg yolk
- 1/4 cup sugar
- 3 tablespoons universally handy flour
- 1 spot of salt
- 2 tablespoons unsalted margarine, room temperature
- 1 teaspoon vanilla
- Optional designs: maraschino cherries, fragmented almonds, and additionally chocolate eggs

Steps to Make It

1. Note: While there are different strides to this formula, this Easter cake is separated into useful classes to all the more likely arrangement for preparation and heating.
2. Make the Cake
3. Assemble the ingredients.
4. Delicately heat the milk in a skillet on the oven over low warmth until simply warm.

5. Spot the milk in the bowl of a standing blender. Mix in 2 tablespoons of the sugar and the yeast and let rest for 5 minutes.
6. With the batter snare connection, mix in the leftover sugar and the vanilla. Add the eggs, 1 all at once, until all around blended.
7. Add half of the flour, the salt, and the lemon zing and blend well. Add the spread in little pieces, exchanging with the excess flour, and massage until it is totally fused. Add additional flour if mixture appears to be excessively wet.
8. Massage until batter is smooth, gleaming, and pulls from sides of the bowl.
9. Spot mixture in a lubed bowl and let ascend in a warm spot until multiplied in mass. (Then again, place batter in the cooler to rise for the time being).
10. Make the Pastry Cream
11. Assemble ingredients.
12. Spot the milk in a pan and bring to a stew.
13. Spot the egg and egg yolk in a medium heatproof bowl and speed until smooth. Add the sugar and speed until sugar is disintegrated and blend gets light yellow.

14. Filter in the flour, add a touch of salt into the combination, and whisk delicately until fused.

15. Empty the hot milk into the egg blend while whisking, and mix until smooth.

16. Move the egg-milk combination back into the pot and get back to the warmth, continually rushing, until the blend begins to thicken and turn lustrous. Cook, mixing enthusiastically, for 2 to 3 minutes longer.

17. Eliminate from warmth and speed in the margarine. Let cool marginally and race in the vanilla.

18. Chill the baked good cream in the cooler, covering the surface with cling wrap to keep a film from shaping.

19. Shape and Bake the Cake

20. Punch down risen batter and carry out on a floured surface into a square shape, around 18 creeps by 10 inches. Brush the outside of the batter daintily with water.

21. Move up the batter longwise, firmly, into a log. Roll the log with your hands to extend it. Interface the finishes of the log to frame a ring. Spot the ring cautiously onto a material paper-lined preparing sheet.

22. Whisk the egg yolk momentarily and brush over the outside of the mixture. Give rise access a warm spot for around 1 hour or until nearly multiplied in volume.

23. Preheat oven to 375 F. Spot the baked good cream in a zip lock pack and clip one corner off of the sack; then again, utilize a cake pack with a 1/2-inch round tip. Line the baked good cream beautifully onto the highest point of the cake, saving some cake cream for later whenever wanted.

24. Add maraschino cherries and nuts to embellish (or add subsequent to heating whenever liked). Spot the bread ring in the oven, at that point bring down the temperature to 350 F. Prepare until bread is brilliant earthy colored and sounds marginally empty when tapped tenderly for around 30 minutes.

25. Allow cake to cool totally prior to serving. Enhance with more baked good cream, cherries, nuts, and chocolate eggs in the event that you like.

26. Rawe Egg Warning

27. Devouring crude and softly cooked eggs represents a danger of food-borne disease.

28. Tips

29. On the off chance that utilizing a bread machine: Use bread machine yeast. Add the ingredients to the bread machine as per your individual machine's headings, and turn on the batter cycle. At the point when the cycle is finished, eliminate batter and shape into a ring, or refrigerate mixture until prepared to utilize.

30. In case you're worried that the ring will shrivel while framing your bread ring, place a buttered oven-confirmation bowl or metal ring in the middle.

12. Buttery White Bread Recipe (Instant Yeast)

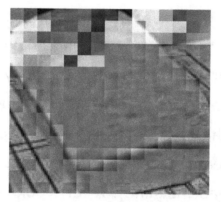

Prep Time: 2 hrs. 45 mins | Cook Time: 40 mins | Total Time: 3 hrs. 25 mins

Ingredients

- 1/2 Cups Milk (tepid)
- 6 Tablespoons Unsalted Butter (relaxed)
- 4 Cups Bread Flour
- 2 Tablespoons White Granulated Sugar
- 1/2 Teaspoons Salt
- 1/2 Teaspoons Instant Yeast

Guidelines

1. Guidelines - Creating Dough with a Bread Machine

2. Your bread machine ought to be unplugged.
3. Eliminate the bread skillet from the bread machine (so when you add the ingredients, they cannot inadvertently spill into the machine).
4. Empty the milk into the bread skillet and afterward add different ingredients. Spot the moment yeast (bread machine yeast) in last and the yeast ought not to touch the fluid (until the bread machine is turned on and the ingredients begin to be combined as one by the bread machine). A few cooks like to make a little indent on top of the flour to keep the yeast from spilling into the fluids or blending in with the salt before the machine is turned on.
5. Put the bread skillet with ingredients back into unplugged bread machine.
6. Plug in bread machine. Enter the "Batter" setting on your bread machine and afterward press the "Start" button.
7. At the point when the bread machine has wrapped up making the bread batter, unplug the bread machine.
8. Eliminate the bread container from the bread machine.

9. Presently go to the guidance segment beneath on "setting up the mixture and heating the bread". FYI - Ignore the directions for the electric stand blender underneath on the off chance that you are utilizing a bread machine to make your batter. Skirt down to the getting ready mixture area.

10. Directions - Creating Dough with an Electric Stand Mixer with Dough Hook

11. Your electric blender ought to be unplugged.

12. Eliminate the blending bowl from the electric blender.

13. Addition a batter guide into the electric blender.

14. Empty the milk into the blending bowl and afterward add different ingredients. Spot the moment yeast in last and the yeast ought not to touch the fluid (until the electric blender is turned on and the ingredients begin to be combined as one). A few pastry specialists like to make a little indent on top of the flour to keep the yeast from spilling into the fluids or blending in with the salt before the machine is turned on.

15. Spot the blending bowl once more into the electric stand blender.

16. Plug in the electric blender and utilize a low speed to blend the mixture. Blend the batter for 8-10 minutes.

17. Mood killer the electric blender and unplug machine.

18. Eliminate the blending bowl from the electric blender. Empty the mixture into a subsequent enormous blending bowl that has been delicately "lubed" with olive oil, dissolved spread, cooking shower, and so on

19. Freely cover the bowl with cling wrap and let the batter ascend for an hour.

20. After the batter has risen, go to the guidance area beneath on "setting up the mixture and heating the bread".

21. Directions - Preparing the Dough and Baking the Bread

22. Preheat the oven to 350 F.

23. Sprinkle a tad of flour onto a huge cutting board.

24. Eliminate the mixture from the bread container or blending bowl and spot the batter on the cutting board.

25. Press down on the mixture with your hands and make a "flattish" square shape with the batter. The mixture ought to be about 1 inch high.

26. Fold up the batter into a tight "jam roll". FYI - Please see the short instructional video beneath for more data on the most proficient method to shape the batter in the event that you haven't formed bread mixture previously. It is simpler to watch and gain from this short video as opposed to attempting to clarify the moving procedure bit by bit.

27. Spot the folded up batter into the bread container.

28. Optional - Gently push down on top of the batter so the edges of the mixture press out towards the sides of the bread container. This should bring about practically zero holes between the mixture and the bread skillet. This assists the bread with transforming into a decent portion shape with no distorted edges.

29. Brush dissolved spread on top of the batter with a baked good brush.

30. Freely cover the highest point of the bread container with cling wrap. Put the canvassed bread dish in a safe spot for an hour for the mixture to ascend into a pleasant portion shape. The mixture should rise marginally over the highest point of the bread dish after this hour long period.

31. Spot the bread dish in the (preheated) oven to heat at 350 F for 37-42 minutes. Wear oven gloves when managing a hot oven. Spot the bread container in the oven.

32. Pivot the bread dish in the oven following 15-20 minutes (to guarantee an in any event, searing of the bread).

33. After the 37 brief preparing periods has completed, eliminate the bread skillet from the oven. Wear oven gloves.

34. Eliminate the bread from bread container and spot the bread on a wire cooling rack. Wear oven gloves.

35. Optional - Brush dissolved spread on top of the bread with a cake brush. This "treating" assists

with making a more brilliant and delectable covering.

36. Permit the bread to chill off on the wire cooling rack for 1-2 hours prior to cutting the bread.

13. Bread Machine Rolls (Buttery Italian)

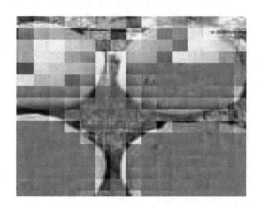

Prep Time: 10 mins | Cook Time: 25 mins | Rising Time: 2 hrs. 10 mins | Total Time: 2 hrs. 45 mins

Ingredients

- 1/4 Cups Milk (tepid)
- 3 1/2 Cups Bread Flour
- 8 Tablespoons Unsalted Butter (relaxed)
- 4 Tablespoons White Granulated Sugar
- 1/2 Teaspoons Dried Rosemary
- 2 Teaspoons Salt
- 2 Teaspoons Bread Machine Yeast
- 2 Tablespoons Olive Oil (to cover mixture before rolls are placed in oven)

- 1/2 Teaspoon Salt (optional - to sprinkle on top of mixture prior to preparing)

Guidelines

1. Relax margarine in a microwave.
2. Spot the milk, margarine and afterward the remainder of the ingredients into the bread dish. You can make a little indent on top of the flour to keep away from the yeast falling into the water (until the machine begins). Try not to consolidate the salt with the yeast (as the salt can execute the yeast). Spot the yeast and salt in discrete pieces of the bread skillet.
3. Put your machine on the "Batter" setting and press the beginning catch. In our bread machine, the working and ascending on the batter setting requires about around 1:30 hours.
4. At the point when your bread machine has completed, unplug the machine and pour the batter onto a cutting board. Wear oven gloves. Sprinkle some flour on the cutting board (before you pour the batter) to stay away from the mixture adhering to the cutting board.
5. Gap the mixture into 12 equivalent parts.

6. Fold the mixture pieces into balls and afterward press them down somewhat into semi-"patties" on a heating sheet.

7. Utilize a baked good brush and coat every batter ball/patty with olive oil.

8. Cover the batter ball/patties with a somewhat wet material to shield from the mixture for dust, and so forth

9. Allow the mixture to sit for at any rate 40 minutes. During this time, the yeast will rise and the mixture will gradually venture into a round move shape.

10.   Preheat oven to 350 degrees before you start to heat your rolls.

11.   Eliminate the cover. Try not to move the mixture on the preparing sheet.

12.   Optional - Sprinkle somewhat salt on top of batter prior to heating. It should adhere to the olive oil.

13.   Spot the heating sheet in the oven.

14.   Heat for 20-25 minutes or until brilliant earthy colored. Preparing time may change contingent upon the size and state of your bread rolls. To guarantee in any event, shading, turn the preparing sheet around in

the oven at the brief imprint. Make sure to wear oven gloves as the oven will be hot.

15.   Eliminate the heating sheet and spot rolls on a cooling racks. Wear oven gloves. Allow the rolls to chill off for 5-10 minutes.

14. Bread Machine Pumpkin Bread

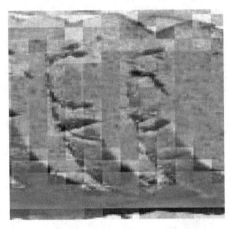

Prep Time: 10 mins | Cook Time: 1 hr. 40 mins
| Total Time: 1 hr. 50 mins

Ingredients

- 8 Tablespoons Unsalted Butter (relaxed)
- 2 Eggs (enormous)
- 1 Cup Pumpkin Puree (not pumpkin pie blend)
- 2 Cups Flour (universally handy flour)
- 1/2 Cup White Granulated Sugar
- 1/2 Cup Brown Sugar (pressed)
- 1 Teaspoon Vanilla Extract
- 1 Teaspoon Baking Soda
- 1 Teaspoon Baking Powder (aluminum free)
- 1/2 Teaspoon Salt

- 1/2 Teaspoon Cinnamon

Guidelines

1. Bread Machine Settings – Sweet Quick Bread, Light Color
2. Softly beat the eggs.
3. Relax the spread in a microwave.
4. Add the margarine, eggs and pumpkin puree into the bread dish and afterward add the dry ingredients. Know that the bread container ought to be taken out from the bread machine before you begin to add any ingredients. This assists with trying not to spill any material inside the bread machine. The bread machine ought to consistently be unplugged while eliminating the bread skillet.
5. Put the bread dish (with the entirety of the ingredients) back into the bread machine, close the bread machine cover and afterward plug in the bread machine.
6. Enter the bread machine settings (Sweet Quick Bread, Light Color) and press the beginning catch. Prior to making this formula, kindly read the tips segment beneath for more data in regards to the sweet speedy bread setting

used to make pumpkin breads. This setting can be extremely confounding on some bread machines... yet the tips area underneath will assist you with tracking down the correct setting to use on your machine. You need to enter the right pumpkin bread setting utilized by your SPECIFIC bread machine model or the pumpkin bread could be under or over cooked.

7. At the point when the bread machine has wrapped up preparing the bread, unplug the bread machine, eliminate the bread dish and spot it on a wooden cutting board. Allow the pumpkin to bread stay inside the bread dish (bread portion compartment) for 10 minutes before you eliminate it from the bread skillet. Use oven gloves while eliminating the bread skillet since it will be extremely hot!

8. Optional - Use a long wooden stick to test if the pumpkin bread is totally cooked. Wear oven gloves as the bread container will be hot. See the tips area for additional subtleties.

9. Following 10 the moment "cool down", you should eliminate the pumpkin bread from the bread dish and spot the pumpkin bread on a wire cooling rack to complete the process of

cooling. Use oven gloves while eliminating the bread.

10. Remember to eliminate the blending paddle in the event that it is stuck in the bread. Use oven gloves as the blending oar could be hot.

11. You ought to permit the pumpkin bread to totally cool prior to cutting. This can require as long as 2 hours. Something else, the pumpkin bread will break (disintegrate) all the more effectively when cut.

15. Bread Machine Pretzels

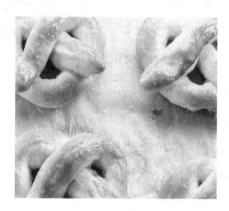

PREP TIME: 1 hr. 55 mins | COOK TIME: 12 mins | TOTAL TIME: 2 hrs. 7 mins

INGREDIENTS

- 1 cup water room temperature
- 1 tbsp. spread room temperature
- 2 tbsp. sugar
- 1 tsp. salt
- 2 ¾ cups generally useful flour
- 2 tsp. dry dynamic yeast
- 6 cups water for cooking water
- ⅓ cup preparing soft drink for cooking water
- 1 egg to brush on prior to preparing

- 2-3 tbsp. dissolved spread
- 2 tsp. coarse salt for fixing

Directions

1. Spot 1 cup water, spread, sugar, salt, flour and dry yeast in bread machine container all together recorded. Try not to blend.
2. Select Dough setting and press start.
3. At the point when cycle is finished, eliminate batter and move to delicately floured surface.
4. Preheat oven to 400F. Line heating sheet with material paper and daintily shower with cooking splash.
5. Separation mixture into 6 equivalent parts.
6. Fold each piece of batter into a 18-20 inch rope.
7. Shape snag into U, take 2 finishes and get more than 1 or 2 times. Bring end towards you, overlap down leaving closes over-hang a piece. Press down a piece where mixture crosses at the base.
8. Plan preparing soft drink water. Utilizing huge pot carry 6 cups of water to quick stew. Add heating soft drink gradually to water, mix to break up. Lessen warmth to keep a stew.

9. Spot 1 to 2 pretzels into water. Try not to pack pot.
10. Cook for 30 seconds, flip and cook for an additional 30 seconds.
11. Utilizing enormous opened spoon eliminate pretzels and move to heating sheet.
12. Plan egg wash by whisking together egg with 1 tsp. of water.
13. Brush pretzels with egg wash. Sprinkle with coarse salt. My most loved is coarse ocean salt.
14. Heat 400ºF for 10-12 minutes until brilliant earthy colored.
15. Eliminate from oven and brush liberally with liquefied spread.

16. Bread Machine Lemon Bread

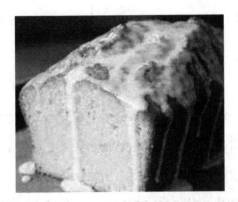

Prep Time: 3 hours 45 minutes | Cook Time: 30 minutes | Total Time: 4 hours 15 minutes

Ingredients

- 5/8 cup (150 grams) milk
- 1/4 cup (50 grams) sugar
- 1 teaspoon (6 grams) table salt
- 1/4 cup (57 grams) margarine
- 2 enormous eggs
- 3 1/4 cup (390 grams) unbleached flour
- 2 1/4 teaspoon (7 grams) bread machine or moment yeast
- 1/4 cup (57 grams) dissolved spread (for plunging batter pieces)

- Lemon zing from 3 medium lemons and 1 orange blended + 1/2 cup (100 grams) sugar
- Icing
- 1 cup (227 grams) powdered sugar
- 1-2 tablespoons (14-28 grams) whipping cream, milk, or espresso

Directions

1. Dump initial 7 ingredients into bread machine dish all together recorded. Select batter cycle. Following 5 minutes, lift top and check batter. It should adhere aside, at that point pull away. In the event that mixture is excessively dry, add milk each tablespoon in turn. On the off chance that excessively wet, add flour each tablespoon in turn.

2. At the point when batter cycle finishes (mixture ought to be multiplied in size), eliminate batter to a floured surface and fold into a square shape around 8 x 10 crawls in size.

3. Utilize a pizza shaper or blade to cut the batter into huge jewels.

4. Plunge every jewel into softened margarine, at that point into sweet lemon/orange zing blend.

5. Spot first piece on its side in Bundt dish. Lay second piece upstanding against first piece and rehash until all pieces have been arranged around the dish. You may need to push them together to crush in the last pieces. Flawlessness isn't needed.
6. Cover with shower cap, saran wrap or a tea towel and permit to ascend in warm spot until practically twofold.
7. Uncover and prepare in oven preheated to 350 degrees for 30-35 minutes or until inside temperature arrives at 190 degrees F. Lay a piece of foil freely on top to forestall over-cooking part of the way through preparing time.
8. Permit to cool for 5 minutes prior to turning out of dish. Turn over so dried up top is noticeable.
9. While bread is still warm, blend powdered sugar in with fluid of decision and sprinkle over the top.

Notes

10.   To set up a day ahead:

11.   Adhere to directions above through stage 5. Cover batter that has effectively been organized in a container with cling wrap or shower cap. Chill for the time being. Around 2 hours before you need to serve bread, eliminate Bundt skillet from the cooler and put to the side in a warm, comfortable spot until the mixture has nearly multiplied in size. Heat as coordinated previously. You can handle the rising interaction fairly by moving the skillet to a hotter or cooler area, contingent upon when you need it to be prepared to heat.

12.   Substitute Mixing Instructions:

13.   Bearings for making bread with a stand blender or by hand:

14.   To make this formula in a rock solid stand blender, add ingredients to the bowl in a similar request. Turn on low to blend until all ingredients are soaked. Utilizing a batter snare, go speed to 2 or 3 and keep beating/working until mixture gets smooth and versatile (around 5-10 minutes). Cover and

permit to ascend in a warm spot. Empty batter tenderly and shape as shown in the formula.

15.   In the case of making by hand, consolidate all ingredients into a shaggy ball in a huge bowl. Turn batter out onto a floured surface and manipulate with your hands until mixture becomes smooth and versatile, an interaction that will probably require 10-20 minutes relying upon your experience. Spot the mixture ball into a lubed bowl. Cover and permit to ascend until twofold. Flatten mixture tenderly and shape as shown in the formula.

16. If it's not too much trouble, note: You can substitute dynamic dry yeast for moment or bread machine yeast. There could be not, at this point any need to break up it. Be mindful that it could be somewhat more slow acting than moment yeast, yet it'll arrive.

17. On the off chance that you just have dynamic dry yeast, utilize 1/4 teaspoon more than called for in the formula. It presently don't should be broken down first; however you can in the event that you like.

17. Wheat Berry Bread Recipe

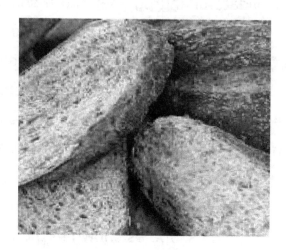

Prep Time: 4 hours | Cook Time: 30 minutes |
Total Time: 4 hours 30 minutes

Ingredients

- 1/2 cup (160 gr) entire grain wheat berries
- 2-1/2 cups bread flour, separated (300 grams)
- 1 cup (240 gr) warm milk (or whey drained from yogurt)
- 1-1/2 (6 gr) teaspoon table salt
- 1 teaspoon (4 gr)sugar
- 2 tablespoons (28 gr) unsalted spread, mollified

- 2 teaspoons (6 gr) bread machine or moment yeast

Directions

1. Bubble wheat berries in 1 cup of water for 20 minutes. Permit to cool (speedier in the event that you add ice 3D squares) and channel. Then again, drench wheat berries in water for 12 hours or overnight. (Mellowed and drained wheat berries will keep in the ice chest as long as seven days.)

2. Add arranged wheat berries to a blender or food processor alongside 1 cup of bread flour (120 grams). Cycle until wheat berries is finely chopped. You will probably have to stop a few times to push the flour and wheat berries from the sides of the cleaving holder back to the center.

3. Join milk or whey, salt, sugar, margarine, remaining flour (180 grams), the ground-wheat-berries-and-flour blend, and the yeast.

4. Select the batter cycle and start. Check batter following 10 minutes to ensure mixture adheres to the side of the dish and afterward pulls away neatly. On the off chance that

excessively wet, add more flour 1 tablespoon at a time. On the off chance that excessively dry, add more water 1 tablespoon at a time.

5. At the point when mixture cycle finishes, check to ensure the batter has multiplied in size. If not, leave in skillet until it does.

6. At the point when multiplied, eliminate batter from dish to floured surface and separation into two equivalent bits. Shape each bit into an elongated shape by pulling batter from the top to the base until mixture is smooth; at that point squeeze shut. Spot crease side down on a treat sheet covered with material paper or a silicone tangle that has been sprinkled with a touch of cornmeal.

7. Cover with a tea towel and permit to ascend until practically multiplied. Preheat oven to 425 degrees around 20 minutes before you anticipate that the loaf should be prepared to heat.

8. Brush risen portions with coating of 1 egg white whipped along with 1 tablespoon water. (This is optional.)

9. Make 2-3 slanting slices in each portion with exceptionally sharp serrated blade or

disposable cutter, being mindful so as not to empty mixture.

10. Heat in preheated oven for 20-25 minutes, or until inside temperature arrives at 190 degrees F, or until base is earthy colored and sounds empty.

11. Permit portions to cool on rack for an hour prior to cutting.

12. Notes

13. To make this formula in an uncompromising stand blender, add ingredients to the bowl in a similar request. Turn on low to blend all ingredients until soaked. Utilizing the batter snare, go speed to 2 or 3 and keep plying until mixture gets smooth and versatile - around 5-10 minutes. Cover and permit to ascend in a warm spot. Collapse mixture tenderly and shape as shown in the formula.

14. In the case of making by hand, join all ingredients into a shaggy ball in a huge bowl. Turn batter out on a floured surface and manipulate with your hands until it becomes smooth and flexible, an interaction that will probably require 10-20 minutes relying upon your experience. Spot the mixture ball into a

lubed bowl. Cover and permit to ascend until twofold. Flatten mixture delicately and shape as demonstrated in the formula.

15. If it's not too much trouble, note: If you substitute ordinary dynamic dry yeast for moment or bread machine yeast, add 1/4 teaspoon more yeast since it is slower. In the event that you need to disintegrate it, mix it into around 1/4 cup of the warm fluid called for in the formula. Let sit for around 10 minutes. Add to other wet ingredients and afterward add dry ingredients. Continue as coordinated to massage and shape the mixture.

16. Initially, this formula called for 1 cup water and 1/4 cup dry milk solids. I have transformed it to mirror my present formula since I don't accepting dry milk. I can identify no perceivable contrast in the end result.

18. Bread-Machine Challah

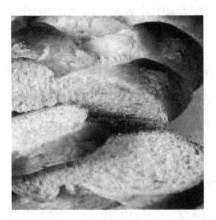

Prep Time: 2 hours 30 minutes | Cook Time: 40 minutes | Total Time: 3 hours 10 minutes

Ingredients

- Mixture
- 1/4 cup + 2 tablespoons (75 grams)water
- 3 enormous eggs (150 grams)
- 2 1/2 tablespoons (52 grams) nectar
- 1/4 teaspoon (7 grams) table salt
- 1/4 cup (50 grams) vegetable oil
- 3 cups (360 grams) bread flour
- 2 teaspoons (7 grams) bread-machine or moment yeast
- Egg Wash Glaze
- 1 egg yolk

- 1 tablespoon water (14 grams)
- Squeeze salt

Guidelines

1. Warmth water until warm and add to the bread machine.
2. Add remaining ingredients all together given utilizing the lesser measure of flour.
3. Select the DOUGH cycle and start.
4. Check mixture after it has been blending for around 12-15 minutes. The mixture should adhere aside and pull away neatly. On the off chance that batter is excessively tacky, add more flour 1 tablespoon at a time. (I as a rule wind up adding 1 tablespoon of flour to this mixture.) If excessively dry, add 1 tablespoon of water at a time. See this post about the main thing you ought to do when utilizing a bread machine.
5. Toward the finish of the DOUGH cycle or at whatever point mixture has ascended to twofold its unique size (open the cover and check), eliminate batter to a floured surface.
6. Fold into a square shape 9 x 14 inches. Cut into three or four strips. Use fingers to squeeze

long sides of each strip so you currently have 3 or 4 chamber molded bits of batter. (See picture above.)

7. Freely mesh strips, tucking the strips on each end under the plait to make a perfect portion. Spot onto a substantial treat sheet covered with material paper or a silicone tangle. You could likewise shower your treat sheet with airborne oil/flour like Baker's Joy.

8. Cover shaped Challah with a tea towel and permits to ascend until practically multiplied. Preheat oven to 350 degrees F around 20 minutes before the bread will be prepared to heat.

9. Brush the whole portion with egg washes (see underneath) and place your oven rack in the lower center of your oven. Prepare in the oven for 30 minutes. Cover following 10-15 minutes, if fundamental, to keep the portion from over-caramelizing.

10. Move portion from treat sheet to rack and permit to cool for 1 hour prior to cutting.

11. Egg wash

12. With a whisk or fork, join egg yolk, water, and salt in a little bowl.

13. Notes

14. Substitute Mixing Instructions:

15. Headings for making bread with a stand blender or by hand:

16. To make this formula in a rock solid stand blender, add ingredients to the bowl in a similar request. Turn on low to blend until all ingredients are saturated. Utilizing a mixture snare, go speed to 2 or 3 and keep beating/working until batter gets smooth and versatile (around 5-10 minutes). Cover and permit to ascend in a warm spot. Flatten mixture delicately and shape as shown in the formula.

17. In the case of making by hand, join all ingredients into a shaggy ball in an enormous bowl. Turn batter out onto a floured surface and manipulate with your hands until mixture becomes smooth and flexible, an interaction that will probably require 10-20 minutes relying upon your experience. Spot the mixture ball into a lubed bowl. Cover and permit to ascend until twofold. Empty batter tenderly and shape as shown in the formula.

18. If it's not too much trouble, note: You can substitute dynamic dry yeast for moment or bread machine yeast. Add 1/4 teaspoon additional yeast when utilizing the dynamic dry yeast. As indicated by King Arthur Flour, there could be not, at this point any need to break down it. Know that it very well might be somewhat more slow acting than moment yeast, yet it'll arrive.

Conclusion

I would like to thank you for choosing this book. These recipes can easily be prepared in bread machine. This cooking strategy may likewise eliminate a portion of the other unsafe impacts of oil searing, All the recipes in this book are easy to prepare and will prove beneficial for beginners. Try these delicious recipes and appreciate!

BREAD MACHINE COOKBOOK FOR BEGINNERS

Table of Contents

INTRODUCTION

Bread making machine or bread maker is a home apparatus for transforming crude ingredients into prepared bread. It comprises of a bread skillet (or "tin"), at the lower part of which are at least one underlying oars, mounted in the focal point of a little unique reason oven.

You can make huge loads of various types of breads with a bread machine like Oatmeal Bread, White Bread, Italian Herb Bread, Potato Bread and even Chocolate Chip Bread! See our rundown of Bread Machine Recipes for huge loads of extraordinary bread thoughts and recipes.

Past custom made bread, you can make utilize the bread machine to make banana bread, pizza mixture, cakes, and so on

You can even make long French bread type rolls (in the event that you utilize the bread machine to manipulate for you and, you do the forming of the mixture and spot the batter in the oven).

It is normally a lot less expensive to make your own bread as opposed to purchasing costly craftsman breads.

You don't need to utilize your oven to prepare a solitary portion of bread. Allow the bread to machine do the preparing while you utilize the oven to prepare supper.

Your home will be loaded up with the tasty smell of newly prepared bread.

Less wreck. The blending and plying are done in the bread machine versus flour and different ingredients spread everywhere on your kitchen counter.

Bread making with a bread machine is a good time for the entire family! Astound and enjoyment your children with bread machine recipes like Banana Bread, Sweet Cornbread, and so on.

19. Soft Dinner Rolls

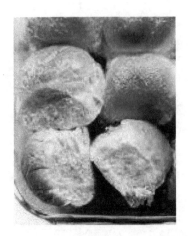

Prep Time: 2 hours 45 minutes | Cook Time: 15 minutes | Total Time: 3 hours

Ingredients

- 1 cup milk, partitioned (227 gr)
- 3 cups (360 grams) unbleached flour, separated
- 1 egg (50 gr)
- 1 tablespoon substantial cream (14 gr) or 1 egg yolk (14 gr)
- 2 tablespoons sugar (24 gr)
- 1/4 teaspoon salt (7 gr)
- 7 tablespoons spread, separated (98 gr)

- 2 teaspoons bread machine or moment yeast (96 gr)

Directions

1. Making the Dough:
2. Measure out 1 cup of milk. In a different little bowl, measure out 3 cups flour.
3. Make flour glue by whisking 3 tablespoons of the flour you just apportioned and half of the milk (1/2 cup) together in a medium microwave-safe bowl. Cook on High in the microwave for 1 moment, whisking at regular intervals. Cook an extra 15-30 seconds, if fundamental, until blend is just about as thick as pudding.
4. Add the excess 1/2 cup of milk to the cooked milk/flour blend and whisk vigorously. It's OK if there are still a few irregularities. They will vanish in the blending cycle. Add to the bread machine dish.
5. Add egg, substantial cream or egg yolk, sugar, salt, 4 tablespoons of mellowed spread, residual flour, and yeast to the dish and select the mixture cycle. Press "Start."

6. Open the top and ensure mixture is the right consistency. It should adhere aside; at that point pull away neatly. In the event that the batter is too dry it might pound against the side of the container. Add water 1 tablespoon at a time. On the off chance that the mixture is excessively wet, add flour 1 tablespoon at a time.

7. At the point when mixture cycle completes, verify whether the batter has ascended to twofold its unique size. Provided that this is true, eliminate it to a floured surface. If not, permit the mixture to stay in the machine until it is twofold, at that point eliminate and continue with the subsequent stage.

8. Molding and Baking the Rolls:

9. Separation mixture down the middle. Structure every half into a perfect ball, flouring the surface you are dealing with depending on the situation to forestall staying.

10. Utilize a moving pin to fold one mixture ball into a 13 x 9 square shape. Coat with 1 tablespoon of delicate spread. Gap into 4 similarly estimated strips long-ways; at that point partition each strip down the middle

short-ways. You ought to have 8 complete strips. Roll each strip beginning from both of the short finishes.

11. Spot rolls into a lubed 8-inch dish. Rehash stage two with the other portion of the batter and another tablespoon of delicate spread. Cover with a tea towel or modest shower cap and put to the side to rise again until practically twofold. This will likely require 60 minutes, give or take, contingent upon the room temperature.

12. Preheat oven to 375° F when you think the rolls are practically prepared. Prepare rolls on the center rack of your oven for 15-17 minutes or until pleasantly caramelized.

13. Eliminate from the oven and permit to sit for around 5 minutes. Turn rolls out onto a cooling rack for another 10-15 minutes. Brush done with 1 tablespoon of softened margarine. (On the off chance that you leave rolls in the dish excessively long in the wake of preparing, they will perspire and get wet on the base.)

14. Notes

15. Headings for making bread with a stand blender or by hand:

16. To make this formula in a rock solid stand blender, add all ingredients to the bowl (with the exception of spread) in a similar request recorded. Turn on low to blend all ingredients until soaked. Utilizing batter snare, go speed to 2 or 3 and keep beating/working until mixture gets smooth and flexible, around 5-10 minutes. Add mellowed margarine and keep on massaging with blender until completely consolidated. Cover and permit to ascend in a warm spot. Flatten mixture delicately and shape rolls as demonstrated in formula.

17. In the case of making by hand, join all ingredients (except margarine) into a shaggy ball in a huge bowl. Turn mixture out on a floured surface and ply with your hands until batter becomes smooth and versatile, a cycle that will probably require 10-20 minutes relying upon your experience. Steadily manipulate in mellowed margarine until totally consolidated into the mixture. Spot mixture ball into a lubed bowl. Cover and permit to

ascend until twofold. Flatten batter tenderly and shape rolls as demonstrated in formula

18. If it's not too much trouble, note: If you substitute normal yeast for moment or bread machine yeast, you should break up its first prior to adding to the dry ingredients. Mix it into around 1/4 cup of the tepid fluid called for in the formula. Let sit for around 10 minutes. Add to other wet ingredients and afterward add dry ingredients. Continue as coordinated to massage and shape rolls.

20. Bread Machine Sourdough Bread Recipe

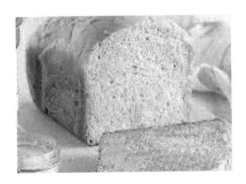

Prep Time: 15 minutes | Cook Time: 32 minutes | Additional Time: 22 hours | Total Time: 22 hours 47 minutes

Ingredients

- 1/4 cup (60 gr) effervescent and dynamic sourdough starter
- 1 cup + 2 tablespoons (255 gr) water (fridge cold)
- 2 tablespoons (15 gr) entire wheat flour
- 2-3/4 cups + 2 tablespoon (345 gr) bread flour (fridge cold)

- 1-1/2 sparse teaspoon (8 gr) table or ocean salt

Guidelines

1. Blending AND AUTOLYZE: Add effervescent starter and water to the bread machine dish. Select the DOUGH cycle. Run for around 1 moment until the starter and water are blended.

2. Open the top and continuously add the entire wheat and bread flour to the dish as the machine keeps on running. Stop the machine when all the flour is dampened. Utilize a spatula to ensure no dry flour is left on the sides or in the corners. Press the flour blend down level with a spatula and sprinkle the salt over the top. Close the top without turning on the machine and let the flour blend sit for 40 minutes. (See the notes underneath on the off chance that you need to put the autolyze, working, and mass ascent on a clock.)

3. Manipulating: Select the DOUGH cycle and let the machine run until it goes tranquil and the working segment of the cycle has completed (around 21 minutes in my machine). Unplug

the machine. Leave the batter in the bread machine dish to rise or move the mixture to a softly lubed 2-liter clear plastic or glass compartment. Cover.

4. Mass RISE: Leave the batter to ascend until practically twofold the first size. THIS IS CRUCIAL. The cycle may require 3-10 hours relying upon the temperature of the batter and the essentialness of your starter. A couple of air pockets will show up on the top alongside heaps of little air pockets on the sides and lower part of the batter (a valid justification to utilize an unmistakable holder). Impact the speed of sealing by moving your compartment to a hotter or cooler area.

5. At the point when the mixture is completely sealed, delicately turn the holder with the batter topsy turvy and let the mixture fall tenderly onto a sodden work surface. In the event that it would not like to drop out, utilize a little, wet spatula to slacken the mixture from the sides and attempt once more. Be patient and allowed gravity to do the vast majority of the work so the air pockets will remain flawless.

6. PRE-SHAPING: Use your wet fingers as well as a wet seat scrubber to get one side of the circle, at that point overlap it toward the middle. Utilize your fingers to tenderly tap the creases and "paste" them down. Move clockwise around the circle, getting the adjoining mixture and overlay it toward the middle.

7. Rehash the interaction until your batter is in a shape that looks like a ball. Utilize a wet seat blade to help you flip the batter ball (boule) over so the smooth side is on top. Cover with a towel and permit to rest for 10-30 minutes.

8. Last SHAPING: (If the batter straightened out a ton during the past rest time frame, refold the ball beginning with one edge and work your way around the circle very much as you did in sync 7. Flip over, cover, and let rest again prior to continuing.) If the ball is holding its shape, utilize your hands or potentially a seat scrubber to make the ball more reduced. (See video) Only do this 3-4 times. Exaggerating this great advance can bring about huge passages. NOTE: If your mixture transforms into a major gooey wreck, almost

certainly, you have over-sealed it or let it adhere to your fingers. Scratch the mixture into a lubed 8½ x 4½ inch bread skillet. Cover it and spot it into the refrigerator for the last ascent. It probably won't be pretty however will likely taste great when heated.

9. Spot the batter with the smooth side down into a lined (can utilize a cloth or cotton tea towel) and floured (I like rice flour) banneton, little blending bowl, or a little colander.

10. Cover and permit the mixture to rest for 15 minutes on the counter in the event that you have time. Something else set it on the right track into the cooler.

11. Last Rise: Refrigerate 8 to 24 hrs. inside a plastic pack fixed to keep out cooler smells and protect the dampness inside the batter.

12. Heat: Preheat your oven to 550°F (or as high as it will go) for 45 minutes before you need to prepare.

13. In the event that utilizing a Dutch oven, see the formula notes underneath. Something else, set an iron skillet on the lower rack during the preheat.

14. Eliminate the bread from the cooler preceding you're prepared to heat. Sprinkle the batter with semolina or cornmeal while still in the bowl so it will not adhere to your material paper. Turn the batter out of the bowl or banneton onto a piece of material paper. Get over overabundance flour. Spritz with water for a rankled outside layer. Cut the bread with a sharp blade or disposable cutter utilizing any plan you like. Do it as fast as possible. The primary slice ought to be at any rate 1/2 to 1 inch down. Make it at a sharp point to the bread on the off chance that you need a decent "ear." Move the boule with the material paper under it to a treat sheet or a Dutch oven.

15. In the event that utilizing a Dutch oven, put the cover on and place it into your oven,

16. In the event that utilizing a treat sheet, place the plate holding the bread on the center rack of your oven. Utilizing oven gloves pour a half cup of bubbling water into the hot iron skillet. Do it rapidly and close the oven entryway as

quick as possible. Turn the temperature back to 450°.

17. Prepare for 32-35 minutes or until bread arrives at 207-210°F in the center utilizing a fast understood thermometer.

18. Allow the bread to cool on a rack for at any rate an hour or more prior to cutting to keep away from stickiness.

19. Notes

20. Preparing with a Dutch oven:

21. In the event that utilizing a Dutch oven, place it onto the center rack in your oven alongside a hefty treat sheet on the rack just beneath it while preheating the oven. Spot the unbaked boule onto material paper on the lower part of your Dutch oven. Put the cover on and place it onto the center rack. Following 20 minutes, eliminate the top from the container. Cook an extra 12-15 minutes or until bread arrives at 207-210°F in the center utilizing a fast understood thermometer.

22. Instructions to utilize a defer clock with the DOUGH cycle for the autolyze, working, and mass ascent:

23. Assuming your machine has a postpone clock, select the DOUGH cycle set the clock so it will not beginning for at any rate 30 minutes- - as long as a few hours. Push start. Watch for the clock to begin checking down. You would now be able to leave until the BULK RISE is finished. You are the person who chooses when the bread has risen long enough toward the finish of the mass ascent. Remember about it.

24. Picking the measure of time you need to postpone relies upon when you will have returned to beware of the batter and what amount of time you anticipate the mass ascent will require.

25. For instance, on the off chance that it is 10 pm and I'm blending the batter so it will rise for the time being, I should add a 2-hour and 30-minute postponement to the hour and a half DOUGH cycle. That implies my mass ascent will begin at 1:00 in light of the fact that the DOUGH cycle permits 1 hour for rising. In view of my experience, I will check my mixture 5 hours after the fact to check whether the mass ascent is done when I awaken at 6:00. The course of events resembles this:

26. 10 PM- - Mix water, starter, and flour just until soaked.
27. 10:01- - Sprinkle salt on top.
28. 10:02- - Select DOUGH cycle. Set the clock for 4 hours. Press start. The machine won't begin for 2.5 hours since 4 hours incorporates the hour of the DOUGH cycle. The autolyze will occur during this peaceful time.
29. 12:30 AM- - DOUGH cycle begins consequently. The DOUGH cycle comprises of massaging which goes on for 21 minutes followed by a 1 hour and 9-minute rising period.
30. 2:00 AM (around) - - Dough cycle closes (blaring may awaken light sleepers). Since the mixture has effectively been ascending for 60 minutes, I have around 4 additional hours to rest and awaken to check my batter at 6:00 to check whether my mixture is fit to be molded.
31. As the temperature of the house changes through the seasons, you may need to change your planning.
32. On the off chance that this sounds muddled, it just takes once or twice of testing to sort it out. The circumstance of the cycles is

distinctive for each machine. Discover your bread machine manual or check on the web in the event that you don't have it. Something else. Analyze until you sort it out. Whenever you have it down, you will not need to reconsider it.

21. Bread Machine Chocolate Bread Recipe

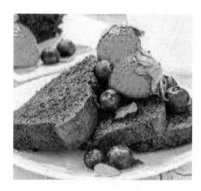

Prep Time: 2 hours 45 minutes | Cook Time: 30 minutes | Total Time: 3 hours 15 minutes

Ingredients

- Mixture
- 1/2 cup entire milk (114 gr)
- 1/3 cup sugar (66 gr)
- 3 tablespoons unsweetened dim cocoa powder (22 gr)
- 1 teaspoon salt (6 gr)
- 2 eggs (100 gr)
- 1/4 cup margarine (1/2 stick), relaxed (57 gr)

- 1/4 cup Greek yogurt (142 gr) (or harsh cream)
- 1 teaspoon vanilla concentrate (5 gr)
- 3 cups of bread flour (360 grams)
- 2 teaspoons bread machine or moment yeast 6 gr)

FILLING

- 1/4 cup margarine (delicate) (57 gr)
- 1/2 cup earthy colored sugar (107 gr)
- 1 teaspoon cinnamon (3 gr)
- 1/2 cup walnuts (toasted) (57 gr)

ICING

- 1-1/2 ounces unsweetened chocolate (42 gr)
- 1 tablespoon margarine (14 gr)
- 1-1/2 cup powdered sugar (filtered in the event that it has protuberances) (170 gr)
- 1 teaspoon vanilla concentrate (5 gr)
- 2+ tablespoons milk (28 gr)

Guidelines

1. Add all mixture ingredients to the bread machine skillet in the request recorded. Set your machine on the DOUGH cycle and push START.

2. Following 10-15 minutes, open the top and evaluate the consistency of the batter. On the off chance that the mixture is excessively wet, add flour 1 tablespoon at a time to get the batter to shape into a flexible ball.
3. On the off chance that the mixture is excessively dry and slapping the side, add milk 1 tablespoon at a time. The batter should adhere aside; at that point pull away neatly.
4. At the point when the mixture cycle is finished and the batter has ascended to twofold its unique size, eliminate the batter from the bread-machine container onto a daintily floured board.
5. Shape mixture into a ball. Separation fifty-fifty. Fold every half into a 11 x 11-inch square.
6. Spread half (2 tablespoons) of the relaxed margarine over the top. Sprinkle half of the earthy colored sugar-cinnamon blend equitably preposterous, at that point half of the chopped walnuts.
7. Beginning from one side, fold the mixture into a chamber and seal it.
8. Slice down the middle with a serrated blade or dental floss. Cut every half into four equivalent

pieces. Eventually, you ought to have 8 pieces from one ball.

9. Move cuts to a lubed 9-inch round dish. (On the off chance that utilizing a square dish cut every chamber into 9 pieces. Or then again utilize a 13 x 9-inch metal container which will hold 16 rolls.

10. Rehash stages 5 through 8 with the leftover portion of batter.

11. Cover your readied rolls with a tea towel, a modest shower cap (my fave), or wax paper. Allow rolls to ascend in a warm spot until they are not exactly twofold in size.

12. Heat in a preheated 350°F oven for 13 minutes or until rolls are somewhat earthy colored on the edges. A fast perused thermometer should peruse 190°F.

13. Permit the rolls to cool in the search for gold 10 minutes. Turn rolls out onto a cooling rack (or serving plate in the event that you are prepared to eat). Leaving rolls in the dish until they are cold will probably bring about wet bottoms.

14. When you haul the rolls out of the oven, make the icing.

15. Spot broken chocolate squares and margarine into a microwave-protected, medium-sized glass bowl or a Pyrex quart estimating cup. Microwave for 1-1/2 to 2 minutes on half force blending partially through to dissolve the spread and chocolate equitably. Keep mixing toward the finish of that chance to wrap up softening the spread.

16. Add the filtered powdered sugar and milk. Mix enthusiastically until your icing is smooth and begins to sparkle. Gradually add more milk if necessary to make the icing pourable. (In the event that you make the icing early, it will thicken as it sits. You may have to add more milk and whip it until it's by and by the correct consistency.)

17. Shower icing over the rolls with a spoon. In the event that you need a neater look, fill a plastic zippered pack with the icing. Zip the sack shut. Cut a little opening in one corner and press icing over the highest points of rolls. (Be certain you have fixed the pack before you begin pressing. I'll allow you to sort out what occurs if the sack busts open.)

18. Notes

19. Substitute Mixing Instructions:

20. Headings for making bread with a stand blender or by hand:

21. To make this formula in a rock solid stand blender, add ingredients to the bowl in a similar request. Turn on low to blend until all ingredients are soaked. Utilizing a batter snare, go speed to 2 or 3 and keep beating/plying until mixture gets smooth and versatile (around 5-10 minutes). Cover and permit to ascend in a warm spot. Collapse batter delicately and shape as shown in the formula.

22. In the case of making by hand, consolidate all ingredients into a shaggy ball in an enormous bowl. Turn mixture out onto a floured surface and massage with your hands until batter becomes smooth and versatile, a cycle that will probably require 10-20 minutes relying upon your experience. Spot the mixture ball into a lubed bowl. Cover and permit to ascend until twofold. Collapse mixture delicately and shape as demonstrated in the formula.

23. Kindly note: You can substitute dynamic dry yeast for moment or bread machine yeast.

There could be not, at this point any need to break down it. Know that it could be somewhat more slow acting than moment yeast, yet it'll arrive.

22. Bread Machine Cinnamon

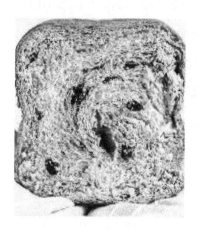

Prep Time: 2 hours 30 minutes | Cook Time: 35 minutes | Total Time: 3 hours 5 minutes

INGREDIENTS

MIXTURE:

- ½ to ⅔ cup tepid milk (114 to 151 gr)
- 2 enormous eggs (100 gr)
- 3 tablespoons mellowed unsalted margarine (42 gr)
- ¼ cup granulated sugar (50 gr)
- 1½ teaspoons table salt (9 gr)
- ½ teaspoon cinnamon (1.3 gr)

- 3 cups bread flour (360 gr)
- 2¼ teaspoons moment yeast (7 gr)
- ⅔ cup raisins, chopped (106 gr)
- *FILLING:*
- ⅓ cup powdered sugar (38 gr)
- 2 teaspoons cinnamon (5 gr)
- ⅛ teaspoon ground cloves (a squeeze)
- *COATING:*
- 1 enormous egg (50 gr)
- 1 tablespoon water (14 gr)

GUIDELINES

1. Add all the batter ingredients aside from the raisins to your bread machine container. Select the DOUGH cycle and press start. Following 12-15 minutes, open the top and check the mixture. It ought to be shabby and adhere to the side of the container prior to pulling endlessly neatly. Make revisions by adding either fluid or flour 1 tablespoon at a time until dough meets this model.

2. At the point when the DOUGH cycle completes, stick two floured fingers into the batter to check whether it has sufficiently sealed.

3. Your fingers should leave a space that gradually fills in. On the off chance that the mixture skips directly back, let it sit in the bread machine somewhat more and test again in 15-30 minutes.

4. Eliminate the mixture from the bread machine to a gently floured or lubed surface. Structure into a ball and smooth into an unpleasant square shape. Cover and let rest for 10 minutes. Combine as one the filling ingredients.

5. Carry batter out to a 9 x 14-inch square shape. Spritz delicately with water. Sprinkle the filling equally absurd. Move up jam move style beginning from one of the short finishes. Squeeze the crease together to seal. Pull each end towards the crease and squeeze. Spot mixture chamber into a lubed 8½ x 4½-inch portion container crease side down or a 9x4x4-inch Pullman skillet. Press down on the mixture to uniformly convey it all through the container.

6. Cover container and spot in a warm spot until practically twofold in size. This cycle will probably take longer than expected (1-2

hours) since it is an improved batter, yet check it at 45 minutes. Utilize a knuckle to daintily push on the portion. The space should fill in gradually. In the event that it skips back promptly, let it keep on rising.

7. Preheat the oven to 375°F (190°C) around 15 minutes before you figure the portion will be prepared to heat.

8. Coating the portion on top just if preparing in a standard portion skillet. Put the cover on if utilizing a Pullman dish and you need a square portion. Heat for around 35-45 minutes or until the inward temperature arrives at 190°F (88°C). In the event that utilizing a Pullman skillet, pull the top off around 10 minutes before you anticipate that the bread should be finished. Utilize a speedy read thermometer to ensure the bread is prepared completely through.

9. Eliminate the bread from the oven and permit to sit for 5 min. utilize a margarine blade to release the portion from the skillet and turn it out onto a cooling rack for 20-30 minutes prior to cutting to try not to crush your portion.

23. Bread Machine Ciabatta Recipe

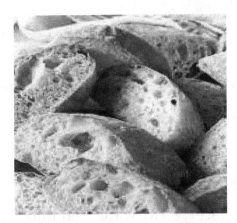

Prep Time: 1 day | Cook Time: 20 minutes |
Total Time: 1 day 20 minutes

Ingredients

- **BIGA**
- 1/8 teaspoon moment yeast (.4 gr)
- 1/2 cup (4 ounces) water (separated or spring water on the off chance that you have it) (114 gr)
- 1 cup unbleached, universally handy flour (120 grams)
- **CRUSTY BREAD DOUGH**

- 1/2 cup (4 ounces) cool water (114 gr)
- 1/4 cup (2 ounces) milk (tepid) (57 gr)
- 1-1/2 teaspoon salt (9 gr)
- 2 cups unbleached generally useful flour (240 grams)
- 1/2 teaspoon bread machine yeast (indeed, that is all) (1.5 gr)
- flour or semolina for flouring the board and your hands

Directions

1. Blending the Biga
2. Consolidate yeast, water, and flour in the bread machine container. (Utilize another compartment on the off chance that you would prefer not to tie up your bread machine that long.) Select the mixture cycle and turn on for around 5 minutes to blend the ingredients. Utilize a little spatula to scratch overabundance flour from the corners into the wet flour combination. Mood killer or unplug the machine and let sit for 12-24 hours.
3. If not utilizing the biga inside 24 hours, place the frothy combination into the fridge. The flavor will just improve - up to 3-4 days.

Permit the biga to come to room temperature prior to continuing to the subsequent stage.

4. Blending the Ciabatta Dough

5. In the request recorded, add the water, milk, salt, flour, and yeast to the biga in your bread machine.

6. Select the DOUGH cycle and push start. Following 15-20 minutes, open the cover and check the mixture. The mixture should begin to look gleaming yet will in any case be tacky. The mixture will twist around the paddle(s). (See video.) If the batter isn't adhering to the sides by any stretch of the imagination, add water 1 tablespoon at a time. In the event that the mixture looks more like a thick hotcake hitter, add additional flour 1 tablespoon at a time. On the off chance that you have gauged your flour effectively, ideally, no changes will be vital.

7. When working stops, eliminate the skillet from the machine. Try not to allow the DOUGH to cycle finish as you typically would.

8. Daintily shower a 3-quart square or rectangular compartment. Utilize a brush or your hand to cover within the compartment...

9. Utilize a lubed spatula to eliminate the tacky batter from the bread machine skillet into a very much lubed plastic compartment. Oil all surfaces of the batter by flipping the mixture over with the spatula.

10. Cover and permit the mixture to ascend at room temperature. Try not to attempt to surge it. Allow the mixture to ascend until twofold. This makes require an hour or more if the room is cold.

11. Utilizing a lubed spatula, slip it under the batter in the corners and lift each corner and each side up and to the center. This is better seen on the video. Be mindful so as not to crush any air pockets. Cover and let sit for 30 minutes.

12. Rehash stage 7. Once more, let the mixture rest for 30 minutes. This assists with guaranteeing a holey surface

13. Forming the Ciabatta Dough

14. Void mixture by flipping around the holder onto a generously floured (semolina flour and bread flour function admirably together in the event that you have it) surface. (I utilize a silicone heating sheet since it's not

difficult to toss into the dishwasher). The mixture ought to be in a similar general square or rectangular state of the compartment it sealed in. Try not to PUNCH THE DOUGH DOWN like you would typical bread batter.

15.   Splash or coat a seat scrubber (or enormous blade) with olive oil. Use it to separate the square shape of mixture into equal parts longways.

16.   Catch the long internal edges of each portion with the oiled seat scrubber and pull it up super about midway and toward the external edge. This leaves more space between each portion. (This is very difficult at the outset, so don't expect flawlessness the initial not many occasions.)

17.   Presently get the external edge of each portion (the one that resembles it's going to tumble off the plate now) with the seat scrubber. Once more, pull it up absurd mostly toward the center of the plate. (See the video.)

18.   Fix and tidy up the shape with a seat blade. Utilize your very much lubed or floured fingers (as though you were playing the piano) to dimple the outside of the batter.

19.   Second-Rise and Baking

20.   On the off chance that you are utilizing a silicone tangle, move or pull the tangle with the formed portions onto a rimless heating sheet. (See video)

21.   On the off chance that you are not utilizing a silicone tangle, use generously floured hands to deliberately move the two chambers of mixture to a readied treat sheet. (To set up the heating sheet, cover the sheet with material paper. Or then again oil and sprinkle with flour as well as semolina or cornmeal.)

22.   Cover the portions so the mixture will not dry out and structure a hull. You can likewise splash an enormous piece of cling wrap with oil and cover the portions with it.

23.   Preheat oven to 450°F.

24.   Allow portions to rest for around 30-45 minutes or until they get puffy.

25.   Spritz portions with water utilizing a splash bottle. Prepare at 450° F for 18-20 minutes. Shower portions a couple of more occasions during the initial 5 minutes of

preparing. Do it rapidly so your oven will not lose a lot heat.

26. Portions are done when the covering is brilliant earthy colored and the interior temperature arrives at 210°F.

27. Permit portions to cool on a cooling rack for at any rate an hour prior to cutting.

24. Bread Machine Brioche Recipe

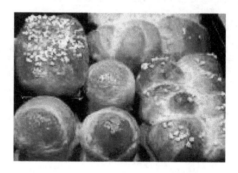

***Prep Time: 2 hours | Cook Time: 15 minutes |
Additional Time: 8 hours | Total Time: 10 hours
15 minutes***

Ingredients

- 1/3 cup milk (82 g)
- 1 tablespoon bread flour (9 g)
- 3 huge eggs, room temperature (150 gr)
- 1-1/4 teaspoon salt (7.5g)
- 2 tablespoons sugar (25 g)
- 2-3/4 cups bread flour (330 g)

- 2-1/4 teaspoons bread-machine or moment yeast (7 gr)
- 12 tablespoons spread, flexible (IMPORTANT) (168 gr)
- Coating:
- 1 egg (50 gr) + 1 tablespoon substantial cream whisked together well. (14 gr)

Directions

1. Prior to YOU START: Set out the margarine to mollify. Margarine should not be warm to such an extent that it goes to fluid. Then again, you ought to have the option to cut it with a table blade.

2. Consolidate 1/3 cup of milk and 1 tablespoon of flour in a microwave-safe holder. Race until smooth.

3. Microwave this fluid glue blend for 20 seconds on High. Eliminate and mix. Spot once again into the microwave for 10-20 seconds or anyway long it takes to transform the blend into a thick "sauce" consistency. Fill the bread machine dish.

4. Add eggs, sugar, salt, 2-3/4 cups of bread flour, and yeast.

5. Select the DOUGH cycle and push start. Following 8 minutes, open the cover of your bread machine and notice the working activity. On the off chance that the mixture is excessively slack, add extra flour each tablespoon in turn, allowing the batter to assimilate the flour prior to adding more.

6. You need the mixture to be adequately thick to hold its shape, adhere to the sides, and at that point pull away, however not "neatly." This batter ought to be stickier than the normal bread batter. However, it should be firm enough for the bread machine cutting edges to get footing as they massage the batter.

7. Around 15 minutes into the mixture cycle, open the cover once more. Start to add the spread to the batter, each tablespoon in turn. Allow the batter to retain each piece of margarine prior to adding more. The batter ought to be smooth and sparkling now and pulling away from the sides.

8. Permit mixture cycle to finish. The batter ought to be multiplied in size. In the event that the encompassing temperature is cold in your

kitchen, you may have to permit the mixture to rise longer until multiplied.

9. Delicately discharge the batter from the sides to eliminate a portion of the air.

10.   Cover the bread machine bowl and spot into your cooler for 6-24 hours. Try not to skirt this part. On the off chance that you don't possess energy for the chill, you should make another sort of bread.

11. Guidelines for forming burger buns:

12. Structure mixture into 2 logs.

13. Cut each sign into 5 similarly estimated pieces. In the event that you need sliders, cut more pieces. You will choose. Make more than one size on the off chance that you need to satisfy everyone.

14. Structure each part into a ball and straighten it to some degree with your fingers on the Silpat or material paper-lined heating plate.

15. Cover every bun with cling wrap and crush it. I like to utilize a straightforward glass pie plate so I can perceive how equitably I'm crushing

the bun. Cover with a tea towel and permit to verification.

16. Preheat oven to 425 degrees F.

17. In the wake of ascending to practically twofold their unique size, press every bun tenderly and equitably with your fingers. Try not to stress. They pop right up once you put them in the oven.

18. Paint with the coating. Turn oven temperature back to 350 degrees F and prepare for 15 minutes.

19. Eliminate buns onto a cooling rack. Cut on a level plane with a serrated blade to use as buns.

20. Molding an exemplary brioche with a braid:

21. Spot mixture on a delicately floured board. Daintily massage and shape into a ball. Gap down the middle. Cut every half into 6 pieces.

22. Pull a limited quantity off every one of the 12 balls to make caps. Fold all parts into little balls. The smoother the better and practice makes a difference. Spot one enormous ball in each form or fill a biscuit tin. Spot every little ball (future caps) on wax paper, material, or a silicone tangle on treat sheet.

23. Cover rolls with a tea towel and permit them to ascend in a warm spot until practically multiplied. This may require 1-2 hours.

24. At the point when rolls have nearly multiplied in size, utilize a lubed thumb or the handle end of a wooden spoon to painstakingly push down batter in the middle (right to the base.) Don't stress, it will spring back once it hits the oven. Brush with coat.

25. Spot a little ball in the focal point of the roll and again brush whole move with coat, taking consideration not to allow coating to pool at the edges between the mixture and the form.

26. Spot singular molds or biscuits dish onto a treat sheet to keep the bottoms from over-sautéing.

27. Preheat oven to 425 degrees. At that point lessen temperature to 375 degrees and heat rolls for around 15 minutes. Freely cover rolls with foil if tops are getting excessively dim. Inward temperature should arrive at 185-190 degrees.

28. Permit the rolls to cool a few minutes. Turn out onto a cooling rack.

29. Best eaten that very day yet in addition great toasted the following day.
30. Forming a brioche portion:
31. Carry out mixture into a 11 x 15-inch square shape with the short side towards you.
32. Move up mixture, beginning with the short side. Separation into four equivalent parts.
33. Spot each move opposite to the long side of a lubed 9 x 5 portion skillet. (I utilize Baker's Joy.)
34. Cover with a tea towel or shower cap. Permit mixture to ascend until it arrives at the highest point of the skillet.
35. Preheat oven to 425 degrees F.
36. Brush portion with coat.
37. Set oven temperature back to 350 degrees F. Heat for 30-35 minutes or until inward temperature arrives at 190 degrees F. Cover freely with a piece of aluminum foil if the top begins to get excessively earthy colored.
38. Allow the bread to cool for around 10 minutes prior to eliminating it from the skillet to a cooling rack.
39. Notes
40. Variety: Sugar-Crusted Raisin Brioche

41. Add 3/4 cup of raisins or currants to the two or three minutes before the finish of the batter cycle. Proceed with step #7 in the overall ways above.

42. Forming Raisin Brioche

43. Gap the mixture into 24 similarly estimated divides after the short-term chill, at that point fold into balls.

44. Spot two balls one next to the other in each cup of a biscuit dish.

45. Then, permit the shaped rolls to ascend for around 2 hours.

46. At long last, coating and sprinkle rolls with sugar and heat as indicated by bearings above.

25. Bread Machine Hawaiian Sweet Rolls

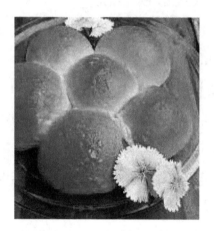

Prep Time: 2 hours 45 minutes | Cook Time: 12 minutes | Total Time: 2 hours 57 minutes

Ingredients

- 1/3 cup warm pineapple juice (76 gr)
- 1/2 cup pureed potatoes (125 gr)
- 2 tablespoons nonfat dried milk powder (14 gr)
- 1 huge egg + 1 egg yolk (64 gr)
- 3 tablespoons sugar (a day and a half)
- 1/3 cup substantial cream, warmed (80 gr)
- 1/4 cup spread, mellowed (57 gr)

- 1 tablespoon nectar (21 gr)
- 1 teaspoon salt (6 gr)
- 1/4 teaspoon ground ginger
- 1/2 teaspoon vanilla-butternut-extricate (2.5 gr)
- 3 cups unbleached generally useful flour (360 gr)
- 2 teaspoons bread machine yeast (6 gr)
- **Coating**
- 1 egg yolk (14 gr) + 1 tablespoon milk (14 gr)

Directions

1. Consolidate all ingredients in the bread machine container all together given. Select the batter cycle and press the beginning catch.
2. Check bread following 5-10 minutes to ensure batter adheres to the side of the container and afterward pulls away.
3. At the point when batter cycle finishes and the mixture has ascended to twofold, eliminate batter from dish to a floured surface. (I utilize a silicone tangle so I can toss it in the dishwasher.)

4. Splash two 7 or 8-inch, square or round skillet with a vaporized oil/flour blend like Baker's Joy.

5. Structure mixture into an enormous ball. Gap down the middle. Separation every half into 10 segments and structures each part into a ball. See this video in the event that you need a simple method to make amazing balls.

6. Spot 10 balls into each skillet. Cover skillet with a tea towel and track down a warm spot for the rolls to rise once more.

7. Around 15 minutes before rolls are prepared to heat, preheat oven to 375 degrees.

8. Let batter balls ascend until about half again their unique size. On the off chance that you let them get too enormous during this rising, they will be dry.

9. Whisk egg yolk and milk together in a little bowl. Utilize a silicone brush to painstakingly cover unbaked rolls before you place them into the oven.

10. Spot rack in a low situation in your oven. Heat rolls at 375 degrees F for 13-15 minutes or until brilliant earthy colored. You don't need them to be sticky, yet in the event that you

heat them excessively long, they will be dry and lose the delicate surface you expect in Hawaiian bread.

11. In the wake of cooling about a little while, place into a plastic sack to keep the hull delicate.

12. Notes

13. Variety:

14. Manipulate a cup of raisins or other dried natural product into the bread batter in the wake of eliminating it from the bread machine for an awesome variety.

15. In the event that you need a round portion, partition the mixture into three sections. Utilize two sections to make a round portion. The leftover batter is useful for rolls. In the event that you're asking why not make a greater portion with all the batter: My experience says it's hard to get an entire portion of that size to prepare completely through without drying out the portion on the edges.

16. Bearings for making bread with a stand blender or by hand:

17. To make this formula in an uncompromising stand blender, add ingredients to the bowl in a

similar request. Turn on low to blend until all ingredients are dampened. Utilizing the batter snare, go speed to 2 or 3 and keep working until mixture gets smooth and flexible - around 5-10 minutes. Cover and permit to ascend in a warm spot. Collapse batter delicately and shape as demonstrated in the formula.

18. In the case of making by hand, join all ingredients into a shaggy ball in a huge bowl. Turn batter out onto a floured surface and work with your hands until mixture becomes smooth and versatile, a cycle that will probably require 10-20 minutes relying upon your experience. Spot the batter ball into a lubed bowl. Cover and permit to ascend until twofold. Flatten mixture tenderly and shape as demonstrated in the formula.

19. Kindly note: If you substitute normal yeast for moment or bread-machine yeast, you should disintegrate it first prior to adding to the dry ingredients. Mix it into around 1/4 cup of the tepid fluid called for in the formula. Let sit for around 10 minutes. Add to other wet

ingredients and afterward add dry ingredients. Continue as coordinated to ply and shape the mixture.

26. Wheat Berry Bread Recipe

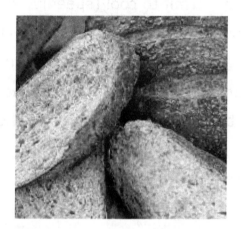

Prep Time: 4 hours | Cook Time: 30 minutes | Total Time: 4 hours 30 minutes

Ingredients

- 1/2 cup (160 gr) entire grain wheat berries
- 2-1/2 cups bread flour, separated (300 grams)
- 1 cup (240 gr) warm milk (or whey drained from yogurt)

- 1-1/2 (6 gr) teaspoon table salt
- 1 teaspoon (4 gr)sugar
- 2 tablespoons (28 gr) unsalted spread, mollified
- 2 teaspoons (6 gr) bread machine or moment yeast

Directions

1. Bubble wheat berries in 1 cup of water for 20 minutes. Permit to cool (speedier in the event that you add ice solid shapes) and channel. Then again, drench wheat berries in water for 12 hours or overnight. (Mellowed and drained wheat berries will keep in the ice chest as long as seven days.)

2. Add arranged wheat berries to a blender or food processor alongside 1 cup of bread flour (120 grams). Interaction until wheat berries is finely chopped. You will probably have to stop a few times to push the flour and wheat berries from the sides of the cleaving holder back to the center.

3. Consolidate milk or whey, salt, sugar, spread, residual flour (180 grams), the ground-wheat-berries-and-flour blend, and the yeast.

4. Select the batter cycle and start. Check mixture following 10 minutes to ensure batter adheres to the side of the dish and afterward pulls away neatly. On the off chance that excessively wet, add more flour 1 tablespoon at a time. In the event that excessively dry, add more water 1 tablespoon at a time.

5. At the point when batter cycle finishes, check to ensure the mixture has multiplied in size. If not, leave in dish until it does.

6. At the point when multiplied, eliminate mixture from skillet to floured surface and gap into two equivalent segments. Shape each segment into an oval shape by pulling batter from the top to the base until mixture is smooth; at that point squeeze shut. Spot crease side down on a treat sheet covered with material paper or a silicone tangle that has been sprinkled with a touch of cornmeal.

7. Cover with a tea towel and permit to ascend until practically multiplied. Preheat oven to 425 degrees around 20 minutes before you anticipate that the loaf should be prepared to heat.

8. Brush risen portions with coating of 1 egg white whipped along with 1 tablespoon water. (This is optional.)

9. Make 2-3 slanting cuts in each portion with sharp serrated blade or disposable cutter, being mindful so as not to flatten batter.

10.   Prepare in preheated oven for 20-25 minutes, or until inside temperature arrives at 190 degrees F, or until base is earthy colored and sounds empty.

11. Permit portions to cool on rack for an hour prior to cutting.

12. Notes

13. To make this formula in a substantial stand blender, add ingredients to the bowl in a similar request. Turn on low to blend all ingredients until saturated. Utilizing the mixture snare, go speed to 2 or 3 and keep massaging until batter gets smooth and versatile - around 5-10 minutes. Cover and permit to ascend in a warm spot. Empty batter delicately and shape as shown in the formula.

14. In the case of making by hand, consolidate all ingredients into a shaggy ball in an enormous bowl. Turn batter out on a floured surface and

massage with your hands until it becomes smooth and versatile, a cycle that will probably require 10-20 minutes relying upon your experience. Spot the batter ball into a lubed bowl. Cover and permit to ascend until twofold. Empty mixture delicately and shape as demonstrated in the formula.

15. If it's not too much trouble, note: If you substitute standard dynamic dry yeast for moment or bread machine yeast, add 1/4 teaspoon more yeast since it is slower. In the event that you need to break up it, mix it into around 1/4 cup of the warm fluid called for in the formula. Let sit for around 10 minutes. Add to other wet ingredients and afterward add dry ingredients. Continue as coordinated to ply and shape the batter.

16. Initially, this formula called for 1 cup water and 1/4 cup dry milk solids. I have transformed it to mirror my present formula since I don't accepting dry milk. I can identify no perceivable contrast in the end result.

27. Cranberry Pecan Bread Machine Recipe

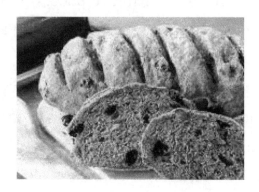

Prep Time: 3 hours | Cook Time: 30 minutes |
Total Time: 3 hours 30 minutes

Ingredients

- Pre-mature
- 1-1/2 cups (180 grams) universally handy, unbleached flour
- 1 teaspoon (3 gr)instant or bread machine yeast
- 1 cup (240 gr) spring or faucet water
- Batter
- Pre-age blend
- 3 tablespoons (44 gr) spring or faucet water
- 1 teaspoon (4 gr) sugar (optional)

- 1-1/2 teaspoon (9 gr) salt
- 1-3/4 cups (210 grams) generally useful, unbleached flour
- 2 teaspoons new rosemary, chopped
- 1/2 cup (80 gr) coarsely chopped toasted walnuts
- 3/4 cup(120 gr) dried cranberries

Directions

1. Making the Pre-mature
2. Spot the initial three ingredients (water, yeast, and flour) into the bread-machine dish and select the "batter" cycle. Permit blending around 5 minutes, utilizing a little spatula to deliberately push flour stuck in the corners into the blending territory.
3. Unplug the machine and let it rest at room temperature short-term or around 8 hours. Try not to leave more than 16 hours.
4. Mixture
5. Add water, sugar, salt, and flour to the pre-mature.
6. Restart the mixture cycle.
7. Check mixture following 10-15 minutes of blending. On the off chance that vital, add

extra flour 1 tablespoon at a time to form a smooth yet marginally crude ball. Add water 1 tablespoon at a time if the mixture is excessively dry and bobs against the sides.

8. At the point when machine signals (if your machine blares when it's an ideal opportunity to add entire ingredients, if not- - add by hand after mixture cycle), add cherries, rosemary, and walnuts.

9. At the point when batter cycle closes, permit the mixture to keep on ascending in the machine for at any rate 30 minutes (or more if the encompassing temperature is cool) until twofold in size.

10. Getting ready and Baking the Loaf

11. Eliminate the batter from the bread-machine skillet to a softly floured board or silicone preparing mat (my inclination).

12. Fold batter into an elliptical shape around 8 x 12 inches. Beginning from the long side, move up. Squeeze the crease together. Turn the finishes under and squeeze together. Control into an adjusted oval shape. See the photos above.

13. Spot on a material covered treat sheet. Cover freely with daintily oiled saran wrap and spot in a warm spot to ascend until practically twofold.

14. Around 15 minutes before the bread is prepared to heat, preheat oven to 425 degrees.

15. Not long prior to placing bread into the oven, sprinkle top with flour. Utilizing a solitary edge disposable cutter (or a sharp, serrated blade); make a few cuts across the highest point of bread around 1/2 inch down.

16. Prepare for 30-35 minutes until the portion is brilliant earthy colored and the inside temperature has arrived at 190°F.

17. Permit the portion to cool on a rack prior to cutting. Or on the other hand cut while it's hot at the danger of crushing your bread. It's great.

18. Notes

19. Headings for making bread with a stand blender or by hand:

20. To make this formula in an uncompromising stand blender, add the advancement (which you made early in another bowl) alongside the extra flour, sugar, water, and salt to the

blending bowl. Turn on low to blend until all ingredients are saturated. Utilizing the batter snare, go speed to 2 or 3 and keep working until mixture gets smooth and versatile - around 5-10 minutes. Add rosemary, dried cranberries, and walnuts. Blend briefly. Cover and permit to ascend in a warm spot. Flatten mixture tenderly and shape as demonstrated in the formula.

21. In the case of making by hand, consolidate the pre-age combination with the excess ingredients (aside from the rosemary, dried cranberries, and walnuts) into a shaggy ball in a huge bowl. Turn batter out on a floured surface and work with your hands until mixture becomes smooth and flexible, an interaction that will probably require 10-20 minutes relying upon your experience. Delicately ply in the rosemary, dried cranberries, and walnuts. Spot the mixture ball into a lubed bowl. Cover and permit to ascend until twofold. Collapse mixture tenderly and shape as demonstrated in the formula.

22. Kindly note: If you just have dynamic dry yeast, utilize 1/4 teaspoon more than called for

in the formula. It at this point don't should be disintegrated first, however you can in the event that you like.

28. Apple Cinnamon Bread Machine Recipe

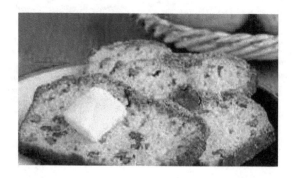

Prep Time: 3 hours 30 minutes |Cook Time: 30 minutes | Total Time: 4 hours

Ingredients

- 2/3-3/4 cup buttermilk or yogurt thinned with milk to buttermilk consistency (151-170 gr)
- 1 egg (50 gr)
- 3/4 teaspoon salt (4 gr)
- 2 tablespoons butter (28 gr)
- 2 tablespoons brown sugar (27 gr)
- 1 cup whole wheat flour (120 gr)
- 1-1/4 cup bread flour (150 gr)
- 1-1/2 teaspoons bread machine yeast (5 gr)
- "Apples in a Bag"

- 1/2 cup golden raisins (75 gr)
- 1 medium yellow delicious apple, peeled and finely diced
- 1 teaspoon cinnamon (2.6 gr)
- 1/8 teaspoon allspice (optional)
- 1/4 teaspoon cornstarch
- 1 tablespoon water (14 gr)
- Streusel:
- 2 tablespoons flour (15 gr)
- 1 tablespoon brown sugar (13 gr)
- 1 tablespoon cold butter (14 gr)
- 1/4 teaspoon cinnamon
- Frosting: (if desired)
- 1/2 cup powdered sugar (114 gr)
- 2 teaspoons coffee (28 gr)
- 1 tablespoon cream cheese (15 gr)

Instructions

1. Dough:
2. Heat buttermilk or yogurt in the microwave on HIGH for 1 minute. The mixture will probably separate but don't worry. Add only 2/3 cup yogurt to the bread machine pan along with all other ingredients except raisins.

3. Select dough cycle and push start. Check dough about 5 minutes into the dough cycle. If the dough is too dry (dough doesn't stick to sides and then pull away), add the remaining yogurt a teaspoon or two at a time until the dough looks just right.

4. Add raisins after you hear the signal for add-ins.

5. When the dough cycle completes, push the dough back to its original size with your hands. Remove pan (with the dough still inside) from the bread machine. Cover pan and dough with a towel or shower cap and place in a warm place for a SECOND rise. This helps make a lighter loaf since bread contains whole wheat flour.

6. Remove dough from pan to a floured surface. (See picture above.) Roll into a rectangle approximately 9 x 13 inches. Distribute apple mixture over the top like you would when making cinnamon rolls.

7. Starting with the long side, roll the dough up tightly and pinch closed at the seam. Use a large, sharp knife to cut the roll in half length-

wise at the seam. You should now have two long "half-pipes."

8. With cut side up, make a snake or "S" shape going back and forth with one of the half-rolls (see picture above) and place into one end of a non-stick 9 x 5 loaf pan (mine holds 2 quarts of water if you want to compare sizes) sprayed on the inside with an aerosol flour/oil mixture like Baker's Joy.

9. Make an "S" shape with the other roll and place it into the other end of the pan as pictured. It doesn't have to be perfect but should fill the pan from one end to the other.

10. Cover dough with a shower cap or tea towel and set in a warm place to rise for approximately 45 minutes. The dough should rise somewhat less than double. 10 minutes before the bread is ready to bake, preheat the oven to 350° F.

11. If using streusel, sprinkle it over the top. Bake for 35 minutes. About halfway through the baking time, cover bread loosely with foil to prevent over-browning.

12. Remove from oven and immediately turn out onto cooling rack. Allow to cool before slicing bread.

13. Apple Pie Filling

14. Combine all ingredients in a microwave-safe bowl and cover. Cook on HIGH for 2 minutes. Allow to cool while dough is rising.

15. Frosting

16. Combine powdered sugar, coffee, and cream cheese. Add more sugar if too thin, or add coffee if too thick. Drizzle over cooled loaf.

17. Streusel

18. Combine all ingredients with a fork until crumbly and the mixture resembles oatmeal.

19. Notes

20. Directions for making bread with a stand mixer or by hand:

21. To make this recipe in a heavy-duty stand mixer, add ingredients to the bowl in the same order. Turn on low to mix until all ingredients are moistened. Using dough hook, turn speed to 2 or 3 and continue kneading until dough becomes smooth and elastic--about 5-10 minutes. Cover and allow rising in a warm

place. Deflate dough gently and shape as indicated in the recipe.

22. If making by hand, combine all ingredients into a shaggy ball in a large bowl. Turn dough out on a floured surface and knead with your hands until dough becomes smooth and elastic, a process that will likely take 10-20 minutes depending on your experience. Place the dough ball into a greased bowl. Cover and allow rising until double. Deflate dough gently and shape as indicated in the recipe.

23. Please note: If you substitute regular yeast for instant or bread machine yeast, you must dissolve it first before adding to the dry ingredients. Stir it into about 1/4 cup of the lukewarm liquid called for in the recipe. Let sit for about 10 minutes. Add to other wet ingredients and then add dry ingredients. Proceed as directed to knead and shape the dough.

29. Giant Cinnamon Roll Cake

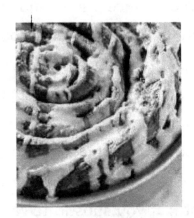

Prep Time: 3 hours | Cook Time: 25 minutes | Total Time: 3 hours 25 minutes

Ingredients

- Batter:
- 1/2 cup milk + 1/2 cup weighty cream or creamer (227 gr absolute)
- 2 egg yolks (28 gr)
- 3 tablespoons sugar (a day and a half)
- 1 teaspoon salt (6 gr)
- 1/4 cup mollified margarine (57 gr)
- 3 cups of unbleached flour (360 gr)

- 2 teaspoons moment or bread machine yeast (6 gr)
- *Filling:*
- 1/4 cup spread (57 gr)
- 2/3 cup earthy colored sugar (142 gr)
- 4 teaspoons cinnamon or Chai flavor combination (11 gr)
- *Coating*
- 2 cups powdered sugar (227 gr)
- 2 tablespoons cold espresso or milk (28 gr)
- Substantial cream

Directions

1. Warm the milk and cream to tepid. (1 moment in the microwave is great.) Add to the skillet previously positioned in the bread machine with the edges set up.
2. Add remaining ingredients to bread machine dish all together given.
3. Pick the batter cycle on your bread machine and press "Start." Leave the top open and check the mixture after around 5-10 minutes. The batter should adhere aside and afterward pull away. In the event that it doesn't pull

away, add more flour, 1 tablespoon at a time. In the event that it doesn't stick by any means, add more milk, 1 tablespoon at an at once "sticks at that point pulls away". (See the photos on this post in the event that you are uncertain now.) Close the cover on machine and permit the machine to complete the batter cycle which will incorporate time for the mixture to rise.

4. At the point when machine signals, check the batter. On the off chance that it has not multiplied in size, let it be and allowed it to keep on sealing inside the bread machine until it has multiplied.

5. Get ready two 8-inch non-stick round prospects (dim shaded work best). Splash within each with Baker's Joy. This has exactly the intended effect when it comes time to get the cinnamon carry out of the skillet. Put in a safe spot.

6. Tenderly eliminate risen batter from the bread machine onto a floured surface. Gap the mixture into equal parts.

7. Fold one-portion of the batter into a 7 1/2 inch by 16 1/2 inch square shape as presented previously.

8. Slather 2 tablespoons of mollified margarine onto the batter and spread to the edges of the square shape.

9. Make the coating by consolidating the earthy colored sugar and cinnamon in a little bowl. Sprinkle half of the filling uniformly preposterous.

10. Cut five bits of batter that is around 1/2 inches wide and 16 1/2 inches in length.

11. Allow strips to rest for around 15 minutes or until they begin to turn into somewhat puffy.

12. Take one strip and freely move it up like a wrap. Get the following strip, somewhat covering where the primary strip finished, and keep wrapping the strip, continually putting the buttered side with sugar towards within.

13. After you have wrapped 2-3 strips, feel free to move the move to your readied dish as it will get hard to hold together without wrapping it too firmly.

14. Keep on enveloping the excess strips by the very path aside from that now you will just lay

the strips into position on a level plane facing the move as you advance around the external edge.

15. It's significant not to extend the batter or wrap it firmly in light of the fact that the mixture needs space to develop as it confirmations.

16. Rehash the interaction with the other portion of the batter in the subsequent container.

17. Freely cover the two skillets with saran wrap and set in a warm spot to evidence.

18. At the point when the batter is practically twofold in size (45 minutes to 1 hour or more relying upon the surrounding temperature), set the oven to 350 degrees F to preheat.

19. Rolls may rise unevenly and be a lot higher in the center than the outside. In the event that important, prior to setting rolls into the oven, tenderly crush on top of the cling wrap with your fingers to push the batter in the center down and towards the edge so the roll is level. Be mindful so as not to squeeze air out. The thought is simply to rearrange it. Try not to stress; the batter will spring back when it hits the oven. Eliminate the saran wrap.

20. Heat at 350° F in a preheated oven for around 22-25 minutes or until rolls is equally caramelized on top.

21. Eliminate from the oven and permit rolls to sit for around 10 minutes. Utilize a plastic blade to slacken rolls from the container and spot them onto your serving dish.

22. Make icing while the rolls heat. Join espresso (or milk in the event that you like) with the sugar. Add sufficient substantial cream to make a pourable consistency. Sprinkle icing over the top.

23. Notes

24. To make this formula in an uncompromising stand blender, add ingredients to the bowl in a similar request. Turn on low to blend until all ingredients are saturated. Utilizing batter snare, go speed to 2 or 3 and keep beating/manipulating until mixture gets smooth and flexible, around 5-10 minutes. Cover and permit to ascend in a warm spot. Empty batter tenderly and shape rolls as demonstrated in formula.

25. In the case of making by hand, consolidate all ingredients into a shaggy ball in a huge bowl.

Turn mixture out on a floured surface and massage with your hands until batter becomes smooth and flexible, an interaction that will probably require 10-20 minutes relying upon your experience.

26. Spot batter ball into a lubed bowl. Cover and permit to ascend until twofold. Empty mixture tenderly and shape rolls as shown in formula

27. If it's not too much trouble, note: If you substitute normal yeast for moment or bread machine yeast, you should disintegrate it first prior to adding to the dry ingredients. Mix it into around 1/4 cup of the tepid fluid called for in the formula. Let sit for around 10 minutes. Add to other wet ingredients and afterward add dry ingredients. Continue as coordinated to manipulate and shape rolls.

28. On the off chance that you need to gather this the prior night, place in the cooler after you have framed the roll however before it rises the subsequent time. Eliminate rolls from the refrigerator around 2 hours before you need to heat them. They should ascend to practically twofold their unique size.

Conclusion

I would like to thank you for choosing this book. This contains recipes which are easy to prepare in a bread machine. You simply have to put the batter in bread machine. You may also choose size of loaf and crust according to your own choice. Try at home and enjoy along with family members.

CPSIA information can be obtained
at www.ICGtesting.com
Printed in the USA
BVHW091720310521
608479BV00008B/1234